D0473657

"No matter how well informed you are, it's not easy to know what to eat in all situations to ensure both good nutrition and weight loss. Problem solved. Heidi Reichenberger McIndoo, MS, RD, LDN tells you what to eat (and why!), in what combinations, and at the right times. Dieting can't get any easier!"

—KATE JACKSON, editor, *Today's Diet & Nutrition* magazine

when to eat what

when to eat what

Eat the Right Foods
at the Right Time
for Maximum Weight Loss!

Heidi Reichenberger McIndoo, MS, RD, LDN,
former National Spokesperson for the American Dietetic Association

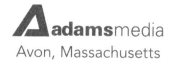

Avon, Massachusetts

Published by
Adams Media, a division of F+W Media, Inc.
57 Littlefield Street, Avon, MA 02322. U.S.A.
www.adamsmedia.com

ISBN 10: 1-60550-103-4
ISBN 13: 978-1-60550-103-1
eISBN 10: 1-4405-1069-5
eISBN 13: 978-1-4405-1069-4

Printed in the United States of America.

10 9 8 7 6 5 4 3 2 1

Library of Congress Cataloging-in-Publication Data
McIndoo, Heidi Reichenberger.
When to eat what / Heidi Reichenberger McIndoo.
       p.   cm.
Includes index.
ISBN 978-1-60550-103-1
1. Weight loss—Popular works. 2. Nutrition—Popular works. I. Title.
RM222.2M43493 2011
613.2'5—dc22
2010039612

The information in this book should not be used for diagnosing or treating any health problem. Not all diet and exercise plans suit everyone. You should always consult a trained medical professional before starting a diet, taking any form of medication, or embarking on any fitness or weight-training program. The author and publisher disclaim any liability arising directly or indirectly from the use of this book.

Many of the designations used by manufacturers and sellers to distinguish their product are claimed as trademarks. Where those designations appear in this book and Adams Media was aware of a trademark claim, the designations have been printed with initial capital letters.

Running shoe and dumbbell © istockphoto / logorilla
Coffee cup and phone © istockphoto / roccomontoya
Beach umbrella © istockphoto / Ju-Lee
Sun © istockphoto / lushik

This book is available at quantity discounts for bulk purchases.
For information, please call 1-800-289-0963.

To Laila and Colin,
who bring smiles and laughs to every day.
Love, Mommy.

acknowledgments

There were so many people involved in making this book a reality—and it could not have been possible without each and every one of them. Thank you.

First, to my husband, Sean, for many extra Daddy-and-kids playtimes, as well as extra help with dinners. To my parents, Sandy and Larry Swadley, for all of the extra overnight trips to Beema and Papa's (not that they minded). And an extra thank you to my mom for offering whatever help she could. To Gretchen, Mia, and Lauren DeMore, for countless playdates. And finally to my kids, Laila and Colin, who still tell me they're glad I work from home even if it sometimes means I can't always play with them. Without the help and support of any one of these people, I would never have been able to finish the project.

To Gina Panettieri, for believing I was the best person to bring this book to life and for her constant help and support throughout the project.

And, finally, to all of my fellow registered dietitian colleagues who were always there with an answer to a question or the ability to point me in the direction of just the information I needed.

contents

part 1

why
when to
eat what

No matter where we turn, we're inundated with people telling us what we should or shouldn't eat. Promises of gaining Superman-like energy levels, melting belly fat, losing inches around our middles, and more come to us via our computer as we surf the web, as we flip through our favorite magazines, in commercials during our favorite TV shows, and between tunes as we cruise down the street. With all of this information so readily available, we should all be pillars of health, right? Unfortunately that's not the case, and a major reason is that much of the information floating out there is actually *mis*information.

This overabundance of nutritional inaccuracy leads to countless problems. In the best-case scenarios, it leads us to waste our time, money, and other resources. In the worst-case scenarios, the advice given can be downright dangerous. In addition, all this conflicting information has left Americans full of questions about not only what, but also when, they really should eat to achieve better health, more energy, weight loss, and more.

When to Eat What answers those questions. It's full of questions and answers about situations most of us face every day as we try to figure out when and what we should eat in various common-life situations. It also delves into the notion of how certain foods, and when you eat them, can affect your weight loss success.

What Healthy Eating Is

Back in the day, the big buzz was The Basic Four. Then there were The Four Food Groups, and so on. But whatever name someone assigns it, the idea is the same: eat several foods from different food groups, such as dairy, protein, grains, fruits, vegetables, and healthy fats, each day to be healthy. And though the amounts may have changed a bit, with today's My Pyramid, the same advice prevails. What is My Pyramid? My Pyramid is a food pyramid that divides all foods into six food groups based on their nutritional makeup. The modern twist is that unlike food guides of the past where blanket recommendations were given for everyone, My Pyramid has a website where you can enter your specific information, such as age, height, weight, etc., and obtain recommendations targeted to your needs. Explore *www.mypyramid.gov* for all kinds of information on the different food groups, portion sizes, and more.

Foods are assigned to their respective group based on the nutrients they provide. Dairy foods are typically great sources of calcium and vitamin D. Grains give us fiber and several B vitamins. Fruits are also loaded with fiber, as well as vitamins such as C. You can see why choosing foods from each group is so important. It helps ensure that you eat all the nutrients your body needs to work properly and feel good. Variety within each group is key, too. While oranges are dripping with vitamin C, bananas are packed with potassium, so limiting yourself to just a couple of foods per group may still mean you're missing out.

The timing of your eating is also important. This doesn't mean you need to drink a glass of milk at 8:05, have some strawberries at 10:15, and a peanut butter sandwich at 1:10. I'm talking about spreading your meals throughout the day so you never go longer than three to four waking hours between meals or snacks. When you eat something within an hour or two of waking and then eat again every three to four hours, you attain multiple benefits. First, you get your body's engine started by giving it the energy it needs, in the form of food, to get going after that long overnight stretch with nothing to eat. Second, a steady supply of food throughout the day prevents the highs and lows—in energy, mood, appetite, and more—associated with a fasting and bingeing cycle. When you go a long time without eating, you likely feel tired and sluggish. Then you begin to feel intense hunger, which leads to overeating, which then leads to feeling bloated and the desire to not eat for a while, and possibly some guilt, and so on and so on. In a word, or three: Don't Skip Meals.

For more information about how to turn these guidelines into real, everyday meals and snacks, check out Part 3 of the book, which includes a two-week menu, recipes, and more to let you create delicious and nutritious meals and snacks that will have you looking and feeling better.

What Healthy Eating Is *Not*

The Ice Cream Diet. The Cookie Diet. The Cabbage Soup Diet. The Lemonade Diet. The 3-Day Diet. The Grapefruit Diet. The Pasta, Popcorn, and Chocolate Diet. It seems like every few weeks or so the tabloids and bookstore shelves are all aflutter about the latest diet craze. Now, while these diets may each sound quite different, they all have two very big things in common: 1) they are all fads and 2) none of them are nutritionally sound.

Many fad diets try to label healthy foods as bad so you'll drop them from your diet. In reality, if someone tells you not to eat carrots, bananas, or some other nutrient-packed food because they're unhealthy for whatever reason—run! To achieve your weight loss goals, you must eat a variety of healthy foods every day. Totally eliminating any one food group is not necessary for (or a guarantee of) weight loss; the only thing you're certain to achieve is a nutrient deficiency. Avoiding an entire food group is just downright unhealthy. And yes, I even mean the fats-and-sweets group. Our body needs *some* fat (not too much) to absorb certain vitamins and work properly.

In addition, while this may sound contradictory, don't eat too little if you're trying to lose weight. Sure, it may seem to make sense that if cutting out X amount of calories will help you lose weight, then cutting out double X amount of calories will help you lose it twice as fast, but don't be fooled. Based on age, height, weight, gender, and activity level, everyone's body needs a certain amount of calories to function. Of course weight loss is achieved by decreasing the calories you take in—but only to an extent. Overly restricting the calories you eat results in a double whammy. First, you become deficient in one or more nutrients, which can lead to various health issues. Second, you just don't have the energy to get through each day. In addition, without the proper amount of fuel (that is, food), your body begins to slow itself down so it can survive on fewer calories. Instead of losing weight super-quick, your body becomes used to surviving on less food. Then, because it thinks you're starving it, it doesn't let any excess weight come off. Not exactly what you had in mind, is it?

Determining Calorie Needs

So what exactly are your specific calorie needs? A registered dietitian in your area can help you determine exactly what you should be eating to lose weight, but to give yourself a rough idea you can use the following Harris-Benedict formula:

WOMEN:

655 + (4.35 x weight in pounds) + (4.7 x height in inches) − (4.7 x age in years) = X

MEN:

66 + (6.23 x weight in pounds) + (12.7 x height in inches) − (6.8 x age in year) = X

Now you need to factor in the amount of activity you do. Multiply the number you figured out above (X) by the numbers that follow, based on how active you are on a daily basis.

If you do little or no exercise	multiply X by 1.2
If you do light exercise or sports one to three days a week	multiply X by 1.375
If you do moderate exercise or sports three to five days a week	multiply X by 1.55
If you do hard exercise or sports six to seven days a week	multiply X by 1.725

The answer you get is approximately the number of calories your body needs each day to keep the status quo. But calculating calorie needs for weight loss requires just a bit more math.

To lose one pound a week, you need to create a deficit of 500 calories. Basically, you either need to eat 500 calories fewer, burn 500 calories more, or better yet, achieve a combination of the two. Cut out 250 calories from your diet each day while you bump up your daily activity by 250 calories. If your current calorie intake is very high, you may be able to adjust your food and activity to produce a weekly two-pound weight loss. To do so, you must create a 1,000-calorie deficit by the same means just described.

when to eat what

Keep in mind, though, as you're calculating and subtracting, that you need to eat at least 1,300–1,400 calories a day for your body to function properly and for you to get all the vitamins, minerals, and other nutrients your body needs. Going lower than that is not healthy and will not help you lose weight faster. To lose weight healthfully, your best bet is to play it safe and stick with the number of calories you get after subtracting 500 from your maintenance calorie needs.

Determining Major Nutrient Needs

Good nutrition is about more than just calories. It's also about making sure those calories are divided up between protein, carbohydrates, and fat in the proper balance. You should get 30 percent of your calories from fats, 15 to 20 percent from proteins, and 50 to 55 percent from carbohydrates. To determine how much fat you should eat a day, or the amount of protein a food contains compared to your needs, the unit of measure to use is grams.

It's easy enough to convert the three main percentages into grams. First, you need to know that 1 gram of fat contains 9 calories, 1 gram of protein contains 4 calories, and 1 gram of carbohydrate contains 4 calories. Next, the formula for determining your nutrient needs is:

$$\frac{\text{total calories} \times \text{nutrient percentage}}{\text{calories per gram of nutrient}}$$

Body Mass Index (BMI) is the scale used to roughly determine a person's fatness. It categorizes weight as healthy, overweight, or obese, and it is used to determine the risk of certain diseases. BMI is based on height and weight and is more specific than using just weight to determine these factors. To calculate your BMI, multiply your height by itself and then divide your weight by that number. Finally, multiply that answer by 703. A BMI below 18.5 is considered underweight, one between 18.5 and 24.9 is considered normal, 25 to 29.9 is overweight, and 30.0 or greater is obese.

Nutrient percentages are 20% or .20 for protein, 50% or .50 for carbohydrates, and 30% or .30 for fat. Here's an example using an 1,800-calorie diet:

PROTEIN NEEDS:

$$\frac{(1,800 \times 0.20)}{4} = 90 \text{ grams of protein per day}$$

CARBOHYDRATE NEEDS:

$$\frac{(1,800 \times 0.50)}{4} = 225 \text{ grams of carbohydrate per day}$$

FAT NEEDS:

$$\frac{(1,800 \times 0.30)}{9} = 60 \text{ grams of fat per day}$$

Plug your calorie needs into these formulas by replacing the 1,800 in the examples with your calorie needs and you can figure out roughly the amount of each nutrient you need.

In addition, it's helpful to know your fiber needs. The following are the daily recommended fiber intakes:

Males 14 to 50 years old	38 grams
Males >51 years old	30 grams
Females 14 to 18 years old	26 grams
Females 19 to 50 years old	25 grams
Females >51 years old	21 grams

Buying Healthy Food

Most of you know that a fresh apple or stalk of broccoli is as healthy as a piece of fresh salmon. But what about all the food that fills the rest of the grocery store? The food found in boxes, bags, and pouches? How are you supposed to know how healthy it is? Just take a look at the Nutrition Facts label . Reading food labels is a very smart idea when you're trying to lose weight or even just eat healthier. The food label is the only clue you have as to what's in a food and what you're eating. The problem is, the government has tried to pack so much information into that little label, it can be confusing to figure out what it all means.

The very first thing you should check as you read a nutrition label is the serving size. This doesn't mean you are limited to eating only the serving size stated on the package, but you need to know that if you eat half as much or twice as much as the label's serving size, you must do the math accordingly on the rest of the nutrition facts' numbers. For example, if you eat twice as much as the serving size, then you are consuming twice the fat listed.

It's also important to realize that the percentages listed on the label—from total fat to fiber—only apply to someone who eats 2,000 calories a day. If that's what your body needs, then go ahead and use these numbers to get an idea of how much of these nutrients a specific food will add to your diet. However, if your body requires more or less than 2,000 calories, you're better off doing a bit of math yourself to keep a running tab of how you're meeting your needs.

Earlier in this chapter, you determined your calorie and major nutrient needs. With these numbers in hand, you can refer to a nutrition label and be able to determine if a food is something you should be eating often or not so often. For example, if your body needs 50 grams of fat a day and you pick up something that contains 25 grams of fat, it may not be the best choice. Using up half of your fat grams on one little snack isn't a very cost-effective way to eat in terms of fat or calories.

I usually divide my daily totals (calories, fat, protein, etc.) by four. I aim for one quarter of my calories and each nutrient to come from breakfast, one quarter from lunch, one quarter from dinner, and the remaining quarter to be divided up between my snacks. This way I have only one number to remember for each nutrient, and it's super easy to determine how or if a specific food will fit into a meal or snack.

If you just want to get a rough idea of whether or not a food is a healthy choice—daily caloric values notwithstanding—take a close look at the percentages on the label; they offer great clues. Basically, a daily value of 5 percent or lower is low, meaning that the food is not a good source of the nutrient. If the food is a low source of nutrients like calcium, fiber, vitamin A, and so on, it is probably not a healthy option. At the same time, a food with a 5 percent or lower daily value of fat, sodium, saturated fat, and so forth may well be a healthy food. On the other hand, a 20 percent daily value signifies a high source of any given nutrient. So you want the majority of foods you choose to be in the 5 percent or under range for the most if not all of the total fat, saturated fat, trans fat, and sodium, but the 20 percent or higher range for several if not all of the fiber, vitamins, and minerals. A few examples are skim milk, original Cheerios, Stonyfield fat-free plain yogurt, and Bird's Eye Steamfresh broccoli florets.

MAKE IT WORK FOR YOU

Though the ingredient list is not technically part of the nutrition facts label, you'll usually find it lurking nearby. This is where you can find out if a food contains a substantial amount of whole grains, and if it's made with artificial ingredients or real foods you could find in your own kitchen. Keep in mind that ingredients are listed in order of the amount included in the product. The higher a particular ingredient is in the list, the more of it you'll find in the food.

The vitamin and mineral percentages given at the bottom of the label are also important to take a look at. You can see how good a source of a particular vitamin or mineral a food is. For example, if you pick up a food that is marketed and advertised as a very "fruity" food and then flip over the label to find that the item contains no vitamin A or C, both of which are usually at least moderately high in most fruits, you would realize that the food may not be as good of a source of fruit as the company would like you to believe. Checking the backs of those packages will teach you things like this.

Know What You Need

In case you're reading all this and thinking to yourself, "I just want to drop a few pounds, I don't need to know all of this other stuff," you're wrong. In order to lose weight successfully and keep it off, you need to understand the basics of healthy eating and how to make food choices that are right for you. That includes knowing what your body needs, when it needs it, and how the foods at your grocery store fit into those needs.

part 2

time
of day
q & a

You've had your nutrition 101 primer, now it's time to get started. Lots of diets tell you what to eat in an ideal world, but whose life is ideal every day? *When to Eat What* helps you make healthy food choices when your day—and life in general—doesn't flow as planned. Making the right food and drink choices at the right time can help you feel better, be healthier, and lose weight. In the pages that follow, you'll find questions and answers about countless eating quandaries many of us find ourselves dealing with on a regular basis so you can choose what's best to eat in any situation.

As you flip through the following pages, you'll notice a variety of icons. Each icon represents a different type of scenario where you may need guidance choosing what to eat. They'll help you identify exactly how eating what, when, and/or how will help you lose weight. The icons include the following:

 for scenarios where you are on the run

 for scenarios dealing with working out

 for scenarios where you're looking for foods to help you repair your system or remedy a mistake

 for scenarios where you need a bit of a perk me up

 for scenarios where you're dealing with weekend-specific issues or issues dealing with going out

 for scenarios dealing with work-related issues

In addition, many entries are marked with a "Morning" ☀, "Noon" ☀, or "Night" ☾★ icon to help you determine exactly *when* each tip will help you get the most out of what you eat.

So now that you know how this book works, let's learn when to eat what!

I like to treat myself in the afternoon with an iced or hot coffee drink. Can I still do that if I'm trying to lose weight?

There's certainly nothing wrong with an afternoon treat like this, but there's a huge difference between a cup of black coffee to get your day started and the fat-, calorie-, and sugar-laden coffee drinks that you can find at Starbucks, Dunkin' Donuts, and McDonald's. Have some healthy alternatives in mind before you find yourself looking over a counter at your local barista. For starters, make sure you choose low-fat milk. Low-fat milk is either skim or 1% milk. You'd think that 2% milk would be low in fat, too, but it really isn't. Whole milk contains 3.25% milk fat, so 2% milk isn't that far from whole milk. You can see the difference yourself:

Milk Comparison (per 8 oz.)		
Milk Type	**Calories**	**Fat in Grams**
Skim	86	0.4
1%	102	2.4
2%	122	4.8
Whole	146	7.9

In addition, don't let yourself give in to too many of the fancy names and flavors listed on the coffee shop's menu. Most of the time, they just mean that lots of sugar and calories were added into that little cup of joe. Also, order the smallest size available. If you're feeling short changed, take smaller sips and savor them to make it last longer. It'll be worth the calorie savings.

Here are a few examples of the differences between various coffees:

Calorie and Fat Content in Different Coffee Drinks			
Drink	Size	Calories	Fat (in grams)
Brewed coffee	8 oz.	1	0
Brewed coffee	20 oz.	6	0
Caffè mocha with skim milk	8 oz.	110	1
Caffè mocha with skim milk	20 oz.	280	3
Caffè mocha with whole milk	8 oz.	150	6
Caffè mocha with whole milk	20 oz.	380	15
Coffee Frappuccino with skim milk	12 oz.	160	0
Coffee Frappuccino with skim milk	24 oz.	290	0
Coffee Frappuccino with whole milk	12 oz.	180	2.5
Coffee Frappuccino with whole milk	24 oz.	330	5

Another simple trick is to steer clear of whipped cream. The extra 80 calories per cup can be a real buzzkill to your afternoon treat.

I'm really pressed for time in the morning. What are some good, balanced, easy-to-go breakfast options while I'm trying to lose weight?

Way to go for knowing you should start the day with a balanced breakfast! Starting the day in a nutritious way will do so much for you. Common breakfast foods include fruits, whole grains, and low-fat dairy foods, which will help get you started on meeting your recommended daily amounts of these three key food groups that many people fall short on.

Breakfast is also the first opportunity of the day to fuel your body's engine with food, and research has shown that breakfast eaters tend to eat fewer calories during the course of the day. Without this "most important meal," you may find yourself feeling sluggish and slow a few hours into your day.

Depending on how your morning goes, here are a few on-the-go ideas for you:

- Grab a banana and 6- or 8-ounce cup of low-fat or nonfat yogurt—bananas are loaded with potassium, which plays a key role in maintaining healthy blood pressure levels
- Blend together ½ cup of your favorite low-fat yogurt, ½ cup skim milk, and 1 cup of frozen fruit—pour it into a travel mug for an on-the-go smoothie
- Try a whole grain English muffin, like Fiber One's or Thomas's multigrain light, spread with 2 teaspoons of peanut butter, and an apple on the side

The key is trying to get at least two of those key food groups in.

MAKE IT WORK FOR YOU

The benefits of eating breakfast regularly are many and wide-ranging—including disease prevention. A recent study demonstrated that eating breakfast is one of six lifestyle behaviors Americans can perform to lower their risk of heart failure. The other five behaviors are maintaining a normal body weight, not smoking, exercising regularly, drinking alcohol moderately, and regularly eating fruits and vegetables.

when to eat what

I love to take long hikes on the weekends. What are some nonperishable drinks and food items that I can pack with me to keep me hydrated and energized throughout the hike?

Like a long-distance or endurance athlete, your body needs fluids and carbohydrates during your long hike. Unlike those athletes, however, your body is using its fuel at a much slower rate. Therefore, you require much less in the way of carbs than endurance athletes. Plus, you have the luxury of time on your side; you don't necessarily need the carbs to be broken down and moved into your muscles as fast as possible. You simply need your carbs to be available for the length of your hike. Fiber and protein are also beneficial to you because they slow the digestion and absorption of carbs and allow your body access to its needed fuel consistently. Portable, nonperishable snacks that will work for you include:

- Protein bars such as ZonePerfect or Genisoy bars
- Air-popped or light microwave popcorn tossed with your favorite seasonings or spices
- Nuts of any kind—peanuts, pistachios, cashews, walnuts, almonds, and more
- Peanut butter and crackers
- Dried fruit
- Clif Shot Roks, which are little, round, crunchy nuggets of protein and carbohydrate

Don't forget to stay hydrated, either. Bring about 1 liter of water for every two hours you plan to hike. That's just over 4 cups. For extended hikes, bottles of water can get pretty heavy, so an alternative to the bottles are hydration packs such as a CamelBak. These are pouches, much like a small backpack, that you wear on your back or place in your backpack. They have a long tube that comes over your shoulder to allow easy access to your water. Because of their convenience and the fact that you don't even need to stop to drink, these packs are a great way to keep hydrated.

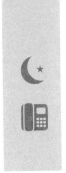

Our whole team at work is staying late, and we're ordering from a stack of delivery menus. None of the restaurants provide nutritional information, so I have no idea what's in the food as far as fats, carbs, and so forth are concerned. What's my best strategy for a reasonably healthy meal with the least hidden fat, calories, and salt?

Your strategy here is to think about *how* a food is prepared and accessorized more than exactly what the food is. Really read the names of the items as well as their descriptions to get an idea of how and with what the food is prepared to help you make the best choice.

Steer clear of the following keywords:

- Fried
- Crispy
- Crunchy
- Buttered
- Breaded
- Creamy (or with cream sauces such as hollandaise, béchamel, béarnaise)
- Cheesy (or with cheese sauce)

Instead, look for items described by these words:

- Baked
- Broiled
- Grilled
- Steamed
- Poached
- Au Jus
- Florentine (which usually means with spinach)
- Primavera (which usually means with spring vegetables)

Don't be afraid to ask if you can modify your order. Even if you're not ordering from Burger King, most restaurants will still let you have it your way—within reason. If something comes with gravy or a heavy sauce, ask them to leave it off. The same goes for butter, cheeses, and dressings. All can either be served on the side so you can control how much you use or left off completely.

If you see fruits or veggies on the menu, as long as they aren't loaded with fat and sugar, add them to your order. In most cases, these will be a great fiber-packed, low-calorie addition to your meal.

Beware of the enormously oversized portions so many restaurants are fond of serving. Become familiar with appropriate serving sizes of meats and grains so that when you order a healthy grilled Buffalo-style chicken sandwich and it arrives on a roll that's as big as a softball, you know that ditching half the roll can help you save a few hundred calories. Another way to handle outrageous portion sizes is to split your order with a coworker. This is great if you're ordering from a deli or restaurant with sandwiches. Deli sandwiches are notoriously enlarged; most are three to four times the size of a sandwich you'd make at home. An ideal strategy is to eat half a sandwich and order a salad or broth-based soup to round out the meal.

MAKE IT WORK FOR YOU

Who cares how large a portion the restaurant gives you, right? You'll be able to control yourself and stop after the appropriate amount of food. Think again. Multiple studies have shown that when people are given larger portions, they will indeed eat more calories. In fact, one study from Penn State found that when men and women were given larger portions for two straight days, the women consumed between 335 and 530 more calories per day, and the men ate between 504 and 812 more calories per day.

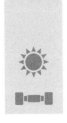

My lunch hour is the only time in the day I have to work out. How can I fit in a healthy meal and some exercise in that short time?

You do have a time crunch, but it's not impossible to work around it. When that clock strikes noon, or whenever your lunch hour begins, you need to be off and running—or walking, or swimming, or whatever it is you like to do. That means whatever gear or attire you need must be at the ready so you can get it on and go. And yes, I would exercise *before* eating. A lot of people find if they try to exercise briskly immediately after eating, they wind up with cramps or an upset stomach.

Since time is of the essence, you may want to pick up the pace a bit compared to your usual routine, to get more bang for your buck, so to speak. I'd really aim to try to exercise for a solid thirty minutes. That's in keeping with the exercise recommendations from both the American College of Sports Medicine and the American Heart Association. That leaves thirty more minutes to cool down, clean up, and have a nutritious lunch.

For both health and time reasons, I'd recommend bringing your lunch to work on days when you're working out. This way, when you're ready, it's ready. No time wasted waiting or going to pick it up. Plus you can pack yourself a fiber- and nutrient-packed yet low-fat and low-calorie meal. A lot of people find they aren't that hungry immediately after exercising and prefer to wait. But that may be a luxury you don't have. Your wisest plan of action is to plan a lunch that has a high-nutrient density. That means it has the most nutrition you can find but isn't too loaded down with calories. You also want to make sure

when to eat what

lunch contains some protein so that when that intense postexercise hunger gets set to hit, the protein from your lunch will act as your built-in defense, satisfying it before it gets there.

Some of the more nutrient-dense foods include low-fat dairy items such as yogurt, skim milk, and reduced-fat cheeses, and lean protein such as beans, eggs, tuna packed in water, peanut butter, and nuts. Fruit also makes a great addition to a postworkout meal. It's loaded with water and carbohydrates to replace whatever you may have lost while exercising. Right there you've got the makings of an array of low-calorie, high-nutrient, simple, and satisfying meals you can have ready and waiting for you as your lunch hour winds down.

What can I eat for breakfast to maximize my workout besides my usual protein shake made with skim milk?

It's a common misconception that people who work out need extra protein to increase their muscle mass. In reality, simply getting the recommended daily amount of protein is all you need and, for most Americans, this is not a problem at all. According to a recent study in the *American Journal of Clinical Nutrition*, Americans eat an average of 91 grams of protein each day. The recommended amount of protein a healthy person needs is about 0.8 to 1 gram per kilogram of body weight. A pound is about .45 kilograms, so for a 180-pound person (81 kilograms), that works out to be about 81 grams. So as you can see, most of us are not coming up short when it comes to protein.

The types of food that will really help you be able to work out to your fullest potential are carbohydrates. Why? It's all about energy supply. Think of carbohydrates as the gas that keeps your body's engine running; they are the fuel your muscles can most easily use as energy. As long as your body and your muscles have enough gas, you shouldn't fizzle out midway through your twenty-minute power walk.

Whole grains and fruits are great sources of carbohydrates. Keep that in mind when planning to grab a preworkout breakfast. To get you started here are a few suggestions:

- Whole grain toast with peanut butter and a banana—the carbohydrates come from the whole grain toast and banana while the peanut butter is a good source of satiating protein and healthy fat
- Oatmeal prepared with skim milk and topped with blueberries—oats and the blueberries are both great sources of carbohydrates while the milk helps you start your day with a bit of protein
- Whole grain English muffin topped with apple butter and a homemade fruit-yogurt smoothie—everything in this suggestion provides carbohydrates to help fuel your workout

- Whole grain cereal with skim milk topped with strawberries—the cereal and fruit provide the carbohydrates for workout energy

That being said, there's nothing wrong with continuing to drink the protein shake, as long as you make sure that you're getting adequate carbs as well. In addition, don't skimp on calories. If your calorie intake is too low, you're most likely not getting enough carbohydrates to supply adequate energy to sustain a good workout.

To make sure you're meeting your calorie and other nutritional needs, keep a food journal to figure out where your usual intake is compared to where it should be. A food journal can be a little notebook you carry around or you can use your computer or BlackBerry, or even just slips of paper. At the end of the day, log on to a calorie-calculating website such as the USDA's Nutrient Database (*www.nal.usda.gov/fnic/foodcomp/search/* or *www.calorieking.com*), and enter the foods and amounts to determine approximately how many calories you ate that day. This will tell you if you should be eating more, less, or the same.

Keeping a food diary is well worth the effort. When you have to write down everything you eat, you're less inclined to grab a few extra bites here or grab a handful of chocolate candies there. That in itself can help cut down calories. But in addition, writing down everything you eat and drink allows you to become much more self-aware of your eating habits. Research has shown that those who adhere well to keeping a food diary lose the greatest amount of weight when compared to those who keep poor food diaries.

To be successful, make it as easy as possible. Get yourself a small notebook that you can carry around with you. After each eating session, write down the time you ate, what you ate, and how much you ate, as best you can. Not only will this help you become more aware of what you're eating, you'll also become more familiar with portion sizes and you'll be able to identify times of the day where eating issues may be more of a problem. Any time you have a problem or something you're trying to change, the more you can learn about the issue, the more successful you can be at changing or improving it.

I try to eat healthy most of the time, but once in a while lunchtime rolls around and it's either fast food or nothing. What are the healthiest choices when I'm having fast food for lunch?

No matter how perfectly you plan everything or how healthy you eat most of the time, once in a while you're bound to go to a fast food joint. Whether time got away from you as you ran errands or you're on the road, an occasional fast food meal can easily fit into a healthy diet. Notice I said *occasional.* The real problem involves the frequency with which people visit these types of establishments. If the guy or gal behind the counter knows you by name, or at the very least recognizes your face, you're there far too often. There are plenty of people who consider a daily fast food meal normal, and that's when the specifics of what one orders makes the biggest difference.

Infrequent trips do allow you a bit more leeway. However, they're still no reason to throw a healthy diet under the bus. Keep your order simple and try to get as many food groups in as possible. If you start with your basic hamburger or cheeseburger, add a meatless salad with low-fat salad dressing. Select low-fat milk to drink, and add fruit if they have it. You'll have yourself a well-balanced, satisfying meal right around 500 calories. Not too shabby for the type of restaurant in which most people get 500 calories in just one order of French fries. Chicken sandwiches could also fit the bill here, as long as you make sure the sandwich is grilled—not fried or "crispy"—and you steer clear of *deluxe* or

MAKE IT WORK FOR YOU

The fast food menu items that seem to get the most attention are the ones with the highest calorie and fat content. A plain hamburger at about 250 calories and 10 grams of fat is never advertised. On the other hand, the super-deluxe burgers of the month—with ads all over the television and in the restaurant—have roughly 700 to 1,000 calories and 40 to 60 grams of fat or more! So if the ads are getting to you and you start thinking one sandwich couldn't be that bad, think again. Your scale will thank you for ordering the burger less marketed.

when to eat what

premium, which is usually restaurant talk for a bunch of extra stuff added to bump up the calories.

The same rules apply to nonburger fast food places. If you're getting Mexican, try ordering simple, soft tacos along with refried beans, which, though it is not reflected in their name, are pretty low in fat as long as you skip any extra toppings such as cheese or sour cream. If you're going for pizza, skip the meat lovers or deluxe toppings and go for plain cheese or veggies only. Limit yourself to one or two slices, depending on the size, and pair with a garden salad with low-fat dressing.

Follow these suggestions, and you can see how an occasional meal from a fast food restaurant doesn't have to spell dietary disaster.

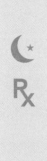

I end up eating takeout far more than I know I should, because when I get home from work I've either forgotten to take something out of the freezer for dinner or there's just nothing in the house to make a healthy dinner out of. How can I have something healthy to prepare for dinner when I get home from work and still have a plan B for those times when I get home and the chicken is still in the freezer?

I think a lot of people end up in this situation because they buy the same assortment of foods at the grocery store week in and week out. You need to change your way of thinking. Instead of buying *food* at the grocery store, you should be buying *ingredients* for a week's worth of healthy meals. It may sound silly—ingredients are food, yes—but an odd collection of random foods don't become meals, ingredients do.

Instead of a grocery list, arm yourself with a menu of your own creation when you prepare for your weekly shopping. Ideally, you should make one big grocery trip per week with a small one in between to restock perishables such as fresh fruits and vegetables and milk. Select a week's worth of healthy meals from your favorite recipes, maybe throwing in one or two new ones a week for variety. You can be very flexible, such as choosing seven entrées and noting that you need seven veggies to accompany them. Or you can be a bit more specific and designate which meal will be prepared and served on which day, including the specific vegetable and any possible side dishes.

The next step is to look at or think about each recipe and find out what ingredients are needed. Then check out your pantry, refrigerator, and freezer to see what you already have. Write down what you don't have, and there's your grocery list.

It may sound like a lot of extra work, but it's really pretty easy once you get used to it. Plus, it's definitely easier, healthier, and cheaper than running to the market a few times a week or dining on fast food or takeout several nights a week. Shopping, cooking, and eating this way also lets you put leftovers to

when to eat what

good use. Instead of occasionally finding foil-wrapped surprises in your refrigerator, you can build meals around your leftovers. For example, you can turn leftover roasted or grilled chicken into a low-calorie chicken salad, and you can use leftover ham to create the Ham and Sweet Potato Skillet recipe found in the recipe section of this book.

So you've planned your nutritious meals and bought all your healthy ingredients. But even the best-laid plans of mice and men go awry once in a while. When you realize tonight's main dinner ingredient is still rock hard in the freezer, your first thought may be to swing by the closest drive-through for a quick dinner. Unfortunately, in addition to satisfying your hunger, many popular fast food choices will also give you far more calories than you need and send your saturated fat and sodium intakes through the roof! In fact, your standard burger and medium fries contain more than 70 percent of your recommended daily amount of both. Keeping a pantry full of quick and easy dinner ideas is a better solution to this common problem. Pasta- and bean-based meals are the best options. Here are some suggestions:

For:	Stock up on:
Simple spaghetti	whole grain pasta and low-sodium pasta sauce
Quesadillas	whole grain tortillas, canned black beans, preshredded reduced-fat cheese
Macaroni and cheese	whole grain pasta, low-fat milk, preshredded reduced-fat cheese
Hearty soup	canned beans, chicken stock, whole grain pasta, low-sodium canned tomatoes

To round out all of these meals, always keep fresh veggies on hand for side dishes and salads.

I grocery shop once a week to save time and money. I'm trying to eat and feed my family healthfully, but it seems like so many of the healthy foods are expensive. What can I eat that's healthy but fits within my budget?

Believe it or not, it's not as hard as you may think. In fact, a study published in *Family Medicine* demonstrates that the cost, per calorie, of a diet based on convenience foods is 24 percent more than a diet based on healthy food. Many of the high prices at the grocery store occur when the manufacturer has done most of the work for you; you pay the price of convenience. If you buy a noodle dish in a box and all you do is add water, you're paying more than if you'd bought the same amount of noodles and spices. Same idea applies to precooked meats, precut veggies, and prepared meals such as TV dinners. In addition, many of us get large quantities of sodium, fat, sugar, and calories from processed foods. By spending a few extra minutes each day, you can save money and eat healthier in one fell swoop.

There are two tricks to keep in mind. One is to try to process your own food as soon as you return from the market. Cut up and wash veggies, portion out meat into smaller packages, and so forth. This will save you time during the week so you won't even miss the processed foods. The other trick is to stock your pantry well. Sure, if you buy two or three different spices and a big bag of brown rice it will cost you more than one of those seasoned rice mixes, but those ingredients will last weeks or months and give you many, many meals versus the one meal the processed dish provides.

A few money-saving tips include:

- Instead of bagged salads and chopped veggies, buy a head of lettuce, a cauliflower, and a bunch of broccoli. You can cut them up and toss them in a colander when you get home, and voilá, it's just like the bagged stuff but much cheaper.
- Instead of buying bags of preshredded cheese, buy a large block of reduced-fat cheese and shred it as you need it.

- Buy lean meats and chickens in bulk and repackage them at home into single-serving or meal-sized portions. Pop them in the freezer and take out what you need when you need it. Boneless, skinless chicken breasts at $1.79 a pound for three pounds or more sure beat the same thing at $3.99 a pound for a smaller package.
- Skip the single-serve packages. More packaging means more money, and it's bad for the environment. Buy a multiserving bag or box and portion out single-serve packages yourself.
- Buy a large carton of plain or vanilla nonfat yogurt for a couple of dollars instead of the flavored, sugar-filled, 6-ounce cups for $0.75 a pop or more. Stir chopped fresh berries and other fruits into it for a more nutritious fruit yogurt.
- Fresh fruits and vegetables tend to be on the costly side. But you can buy by the season to save money and supplement with canned or frozen fruits and vegetables that are packaged without any additional sauces or seasonings.

You can see how cheaper shopping and healthier shopping almost go hand in hand when you can take a little extra time and do more of the work yourself.

My doctor told me my blood sugar is a bit high and I need to lose weight to help keep me from getting Type 2 diabetes. I thought fruit would be a good snack, but some friends said I shouldn't eat fruit if my blood sugar is high. Is that true? Can I eat fruit? If so, how much, and is there a time that's best?

There are very few, if any, reasons why a person should not eat fruit—and high blood sugar levels are certainly not one of them. However, because fruit does have a high content of a quickly absorbed type of sugar called *fructose*, it is important not to eat too much at once. When you eat it is also key.

When choosing your fruit, be sure to pick something that contains fiber to help slow the absorption of the sugar. All varieties of whole fruit contain fiber (the amount varies from fruit to fruit)—but fruit juice, even 100% fruit juice, does not. Limit your choices to only whole fruit and stay away from fruit juice. In addition, stay away from canned fruit that contains heavy syrup. Select canned fruits that are packed in juice and/or say *No Sugar Added* on the label.

As far as the amount of fruit to eat, stick to one serving at a time and aim for three servings over the course of the day. A serving varies from fruit to fruit. For canned fruit, just check the label. But fresh fruit requires a bit more thought. For most fruits, a serving is considered one medium fruit, such as one medium apple, pear, or orange. One exception to this rule is bananas, in which case half a banana is considered a serving. For small fruits, such as berries or grapes, or fruits that are typically cut up, such as melon, one serving is ½ cup. Dried fruits are also an option, but they tend to be more of a concentrated source of sugar. A serving of dried fruit is 2 tablespoons.

Due to the rapid absorption of the sugar found in fruit, anyone with blood sugar concerns should be sure to eat sugar with a meal or, at the very least, with a protein- and/or fiber-rich snack. This slows the absorption of the sugar, which reduces the elevation of the blood sugar. Having a serving of fruit immediately after lunch would be perfect, as would incorporating a serving of fruit into your dinner. As far as snacks go, there is nothing wrong with a snack of fruit, but you

when to eat what

need to be a bit more creative in how to fit it in. Pair a pear with some reduced-fat cheese, for example, or munch on grapes *and* nuts. The only time I wouldn't eat fruit would be right before bed. If the fruit did cause a rise in your blood sugar, this rise could possibly be followed by a drop during the night while you were sleeping. You wouldn't be aware of the symptoms or be able to do anything to alleviate the problem.

I actually love to eat salads, but I want them to be as nutritionally beneficial as possible. How should I build my salad?

A big healthy salad filled with loads of veggies and a bit of lean protein can make a fantastic lunch. The veggies are full of vitamins as well as fiber, which can help keep you full longer and prevent those feelings of never-ending hunger, which can lead to munching all day. A lean protein component such as boiled eggs, tuna, grilled chicken, or beans can also help provide immediate as well as lasting satiety.

One of the keys to a healthy salad is forming a good base. Choosing a nutrient-packed lettuce can be the difference between a powerhouse of a salad or a just okay lunch. It used to be a salad was iceberg lettuce with a few tomato slices, but then some people started adding things like raw spinach. Now it's common to find an assortment of greens in your favorite salad bar or the produce department of your local grocery store. Yes, these choices make ordering or creating a salad that much more complicated, but today's salads are much more nutritious. Iceberg, once the star of the show, is now the black sheep of the lettuce family; it certainly lacks the nutritional punch that other greens provide. Iceberg *is* full of water and it does add a refreshing crunch to any salad, which are enough reasons for me to include it as one of a salad's leafy starters, but for real nutrition you're wise to want to mix in some more greenery. When it comes to most foods, the darker the color the better, and the same principle applies to lettuces and greens. This puts romaine lettuce and spinach at the top of the list, nutritionally speaking. You can see how they compare when you look at how much of the daily recommended amount 1 cup of each provides:

Type of Greens	Vitamin C	Vitamin A	Folic Acid	Vitamin K
Romaine	19%	82%	16%	46%
Spinach	14%	56%	15%	138%
Iceberg	3%	7%	5%	16%

when to eat *what*

How you dress your salad can also make a big nutritional difference. Many people opt for a fat-free salad dressing, but doing so may mean they miss out on many of the valuable salad nutrients. Many of the vitamins in common salad fixings are fat soluble. That means they need fat in order to be absorbed. By topping the salad with a fat-free dressing, that much needed fat source is missing. This is true especially in situations where the salad is the meal and no more fat sources are to be eaten. To keep calories in check but still get your nutrients, choose a full-fat or even reduced-fat dressing and limit the amount. A good technique is to have the dressing on the side and dip each bite into it. This way each forkful gets a taste but the salad isn't drowning in dressing.

I work out in the morning but can't start my day without my coffee. Is it okay to drink coffee before exercising?

Definitely. In fact, many athletes do so regularly. When researchers studied the subject they found that not only is coffee fine to drink before working out, it's also helpful to a workout. The researchers had participants drink a moderate amount of coffee before they worked out. What they found was that the coffee drinkers in the study actually performed better in their workout. What was even more interesting, though, was that they felt as though they hadn't worked as hard as they usually did. You see, coffee, or more specifically the caffeine in coffee, is a stimulant—and it does more than just stimulate your mind to wake you up in the morning; it can actually stimulate your body to work a bit faster. In fact, caffeine is one of the most commonly used stimulants by athletes. It's allowed by organizations such as the National Collegiate Athletic Association (NCAA), but athletes must keep the concentration of caffeine in their urine below 15 micrograms per milliliter to participate in their sport.

However, due to its stimulating properties, you should not drink too much before undertaking an activity that increases your heart rate itself. The side effects of too much caffeine can be insomnia, nervousness, restlessness, increased heart rate, and stomach irritation. Keep in mind, too, that coffee may not be your only source of caffeine; you may be ingesting it from other beverages, foods, and supplements. Other common sources of caffeine are tea, soda, chocolate, and guarana.

MAKE IT WORK FOR YOU

Coffee seems to be in and out of the news often. One week it's good, the next week it's bad. It's hard to keep it all straight. But the results of a large study at Harvard School of Public Health are quite convincing regarding the positive effects of coffee. They followed almost 42,000 men for twelve years and more than 84,000 women for eighteen years. They found that those who drank the most coffee had a much lower risk of developing Type 2 diabetes. While both caffeinated and decaffeinated coffee lowered the risk of the disease, the caffeinated coffee seemed to lower one's risk much more.

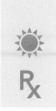

Whoever suggested soup for lunch as a low-calorie solution didn't try making it through the afternoon on just soup! It's 90 percent water. Are there varieties of soup that really feel like a meal?

The fact that soup is so full of water is a blessing and a curse. It can be a great low-calorie lunch option, but many soups may actually be too low in calories to count as an adequate meal. To make your soup du jour more satisfying, look for soups that are bean based—lentil, split pea, black bean. The fiber and protein in the beans really boost the staying power of the meal.

You can also use soup as your lunch's appetizer. Studies have shown that when you eat soup before your meal, you end up consuming fewer calories at that meal. In the studies, they use clear, broth-based soups that can be filled with beans, lean meats, and/or vegetables. Stay away from chowders and other creamy soups that are loaded with calories. Consider packing half a sandwich or a small grilled chicken salad to enjoy with your hot bowl of soup. Both of these items will add more substance and satiety-fueling protein and fiber to your lunch but won't overwhelm your body with extra calories.

MAKE IT WORK FOR YOU

Many canned soups are loaded with sodium. In fact, it wouldn't be difficult at all to find a soup with nearly a day's worth of sodium in just one can. Low-sodium soups do exist, they're just a little trickier to find sometimes. Search on the upper or lower shelves and at healthier markets like Whole Foods. You could also take a couple of hours on the weekend and make a big pot of your favorite vegetarian chili or lentil soup. Just freeze it in individual containers and you have several ready-to-go lunches.

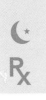

I often have trouble falling asleep at night. Is there something I can eat or drink before bedtime to help me sleep?

If you're looking for a good night's sleep, you should first try drinking an old-fashioned glass of warm milk. Warm or not, milk is a great source of the amino acid tryptophan, which many studies have shown can help improve sleep—especially in people who have trouble sleeping. Tryptophan is a precursor to the chemical serotonin, whose job is to slow down a lot of the action going on in your brain so you can wind down and go to sleep. It's also a precursor to melatonin, another substance that helps induce sleep. If you're not crazy about drinking milk, try drinking cherry juice. Tart Montmorency cherries are one of the best sources of melatonin in the diet.

Carbohydrates can also help lull you to dreamland, especially when eaten with tryptophan-containing foods. When you put it all together, some examples of preslumber snacks are:

- Whole grain graham crackers with warm milk
- A bowl of oatmeal made with skim or 1% milk
- Nonfat or low-fat yogurt with some whole grain cereal mixed into it
- Whole grain toast with cherry juice
- Nonfat or low-fat yogurt with fruit

If you're having problems sleeping, there are also some foods and meals you may want to avoid. Just as carbohydrates can lead to a better night's sleep, protein and fat-rich meals—especially those containing little or no carbohydrates—do the opposite. They help keep the brain action jumping, making relaxing and falling to sleep more difficult.

MAKE IT WORK FOR YOU

If plain milk is a bit too bland for you, try adding a few squirts of one of the flavorings used in making flavored coffees, a drop of your favorite extract, or a couple spoonfuls of the popular flavored nondairy creamers. You can create all types of milk concoctions, including hazelnut, peppermint, Irish cream, vanilla, almond, and more.

when to eat what

In addition, large meals may keep you from falling asleep. They take much longer to digest, which means your body remains active and takes longer to slow down.

Highly spiced foods—as well as gas-producing foods such as beans and cruciferous veggies like broccoli, cauliflower, and cabbage—may cause discomfort, which can make falling asleep difficult, too.

While there are a couple of drinks that will help you get some zzzz's, there are also drinks you should avoid. While it may seem like common sense not to drink coffee before going to bed, don't forget to avoid other caffeine-containing beverages in the evening, too. Mugs of hot chocolate and hot tea (decaf notwithstanding) may seem relaxing in the moment, but they are sources of caffeine and can keep you awake. Other beverages and snacks that may have hidden caffeine are shown in the table on the following page.

MAKE IT WORK FOR YOU

Getting adequate sleep may do more for you than just make you feel more awake during the day. Researchers in Boston found that when workers were well rested they made healthier food choices. Poor food choices, no matter what the cause, can lead to weight gain—or at the very least, make losing weight much more difficult. If that's not enough incentive to hit the sack a little earlier, know that the researchers also found that the workers who had the healthy sleep patterns actually enjoyed their jobs better and reported less stress.

Average Caffeine Content of Various Drinks and Foods		
Drink	Size	Caffeine (in milligrams)
Arizona Iced Tea	12 oz.	26
Hot chocolate	8 oz.	9
Cola	12 oz.	54
Jolt	12 oz.	72
Mountain Dew	12 oz.	54
ROCKSTAR energy drink	16 oz.	80
Hershey's Special Dark chocolate	1.45 oz.	31
Hershey's Kisses	9	9

Alcohol, believe it or not, can keep you awake as well. While it may seem like having a few drinks helps you unwind and sleep better, it's actually not a truly restful sleep, so you'll probably end up still feeling tired once you wake up.

If I don't exercise in the morning, I won't do it at all. Eating breakfast before a workout doesn't sit well, but skipping breakfast causes me to lose steam before I'm done at the gym. What can I eat that's light enough so it won't feel like a lump in my stomach but will let me get through my routine?

Your best bet is to divide breakfast into two small snacks: one before your workout to give your muscles the energy they need, and the second after your workout to restore what you've just used up and to get you through the rest of the morning.

Most sports nutritionists recommend that you eat within an hour of your activity. The most important nutrients your body needs to work out to its best ability are simple carbohydrates. Water and fruits fit the bill perfectly. Fruits are full of easily digestible and useable simple carbohydrates, and they are also full of water. Assuming you're exercising moderately, say thirty to sixty minutes, you should do fine with a small serving of fruit. In addition, hydrate yourself during your workout as needed. A few sips every five or ten minutes should be plenty if you're exercising moderately.

Once you're done with your workout, you need to restore all those energy reserves your body just used up, plus you need to be able to make it to lunch. Your second breakfast should be a three-parter. First, you want fluids to replace what you lost in sweat; water or 100% juice are ideal choices. You also want carbohydrates to replace

MAKE IT WORK FOR YOU

Breakfast gives you a great opportunity to start meeting your body's daily requirements of fruit. Fruits are filled with fiber, vitamins, and minerals yet are low in the nutrients you should limit such as calories, fat, and sodium. The specific combination of nutrients that are found in (as well as those missing from) fruits make them ideal in preventing countless diseases and health conditions. In fact, it's been shown in research that eating at least three servings of fruit each day can help protect you from developing age-related macular degeneration, the leading cause of blindness in older Americans.

all the energy stores you used up exercising, and some protein to satisfy you now and keep you satisfied until your next meal.

Here's one approximate pattern to follow:

Pre Workout: 1 to 2 cups fresh fruit, water

During Workout: work out for 40 minutes; sip water every five to ten minutes

Post Workout: 8 ounces 100% orange juice, 1 to 2 slices whole grain toast with 1 teaspoon of peanut butter per slice, an 8-ounce glass of skim milk

I know that fruit is good for me, but I don't really like it. I try to drink fruit juice instead. Is fruit juice a good replacement for actual fruit?

First, let's talk about the difference between fruit *drinks* and fruit *juice*. There seems to be a common misconception out there that all fruit drinks are juice and therefore must be a healthy beverage choice. Unfortunately, it's not true. The closest many fruit drinks come to containing fruit is the fruit flavoring that's added. Some contain only 10 percent real fruit juice. What this means is that 90 to 100 percent of these "fruit" drinks are really just liquid sugar. If you're looking for a serving of vitamin-containing real fruit, then only consume drinks that state they are 100% fruit juice. Those are the magic words. Also, make sure these drinks have no added sugar.

That being said, even 100% fruit juice isn't something you want to be guzzling 24 hours a day. Even though it is made from real fruit with no added sugar, fruit and its juices naturally contain sugar and it's the simple, quickly absorbed kind. And this sugar doesn't come free. Just 1 cup of 100% fruit juice can contain anywhere from 110 to 170 calories. And before you think those bottles of juice you find in the convenience store coolers are one serving, think again. Many contain at least two servings, so we're talking at least 200 to 300 (or more!) calories.

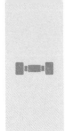

I'm doing a marathon walk (26.2 miles) and will be out on the course for hours. I don't want to get hungry or dehydrated, but I also don't want to eat too much and cramp up. When should I eat and what?

A marathon walk (and even the training) are certainly endurance events. Studies have shown that to replenish after exercising, especially intense events, the most important components are fluids, electrolytes, and carbohydrates. For an activity that lasts for an extended period of time, you should look at eating and drinking as a continual refueling. Your body stores extra glucose (sugar) or energy as glycogen and only so much of it can be stored. The same goes for fluids. A long as you keep using these up, you must keep replacing them so you have enough of these nutrients for your body to make it through the long walk.

Your challenge, obviously, is that your sources of these nutrients need to be as portable as possible. Fortunately, there is no shortage of sources of carbohydrates that are small, simple to carry, and easy to eat, digest, and use—including gels, pastes, bars, and even jellybeans. You must also consider the amount you need. Of course, part of this involves trial and error on what your body needs and what may be too much. Some options may make you feel unwell, or they will not energize you enough compared to a different style of fuel. Some people find the bars a bit dry while others find the jellybeans too sweet. But no matter your personal taste, aim to get about 30 to 60 grams of simple, easily digestible carbohydrate every hour of the walk. Avoid protein fiber and fat; these will slow the absorption and not allow your body to get and use the energy as quickly as possible. Some portable simple carb snacks, along with their carbohydrate content, include:

when to eat *what*

Snack	Carbohydrates (in grams)
1 small banana	30
1 medium apple, peeled	16
1 fruit-and-cereal bar	26
1 CLIF BAR	41
1 Luna Bar	26
1 PowerBar	17
1 oz. Jelly Belly Sports Beans	24
1 GU Energy Gel	25
1 PowerBar Gel	27
1 CLIF SHOT Energy Gel	25
4 GU Energy Chews	23
1 package Sharkies Organic Energy Sports Chews	36
3 CLIF SHOT Bloks	24

As I mentioned, fluid and electrolytes must be continually replaced as well; for an activity of this length, afterwards is not the only time you want to think about fluids. Two hours prior to the start you should drink about 2 cups of fluid, followed by 1 cup about fifteen minutes before. Continue to hydrate during the walk by drinking 5 to 12 ounces of fluids every fifteen minutes for the length of the event.

For short-term bouts of exercise, water is usually the preferred replacement. But for activities lasting longer than an hour—for which a marathon or even half-marathon walk certainly qualifies—water doesn't cut it. Traditionally in these situations, a sports drink such as Gatorade, Powerade, or something similar is the beverage of choice. But new research is showing that another, far yummier drink is just as beneficial. In an Indiana University study, cyclists who drank chocolate milk did equally as well as those who drank a carbohydrate-based sports drink when it came to how long they were able to work out and the total amount of work they were actually able to perform.

Chocolate milk contains the carbohydrates necessary to help your muscles recover and to provide spurts of energy as your body continues to work out. Also, along with the fluids chocolate milk can give your body, it contains the needed electrolytes to keep systems in your body balanced and functioning properly. Plus, it's cheaper than many sports drinks. Yes, carrying around a gallon of chocolate milk isn't really going to work during a marathon walk, but as luck would have it, in recent years we've started to see single-serving, no-refrigeration-necessary milk boxes appearing on supermarket shelves. Similar to juice boxes, they can fit perfectly in a small pack while on a long walk.

If you decide to go the chocolate milk route, you should know that not all chocolate milk is created equal. When you're involved in an intense exercise event, the type of milk you choose is of lesser importance. But on a day-to-day basis, you need to be a bit more careful. One cup of skim milk and 1 tablespoon of chocolate syrup contains about 130 calories, 20 grams of sugar, and no fat. However, it's easy to buy ready-to-drink chocolate milk that contains close to 200 calories, almost 30 grams (7 teaspoons!) of sugar, and several grams of fat. When you also consider that many of the individual containers of chocolate milk actually contain two servings, this means drinking one bottle is like eating half a medium-sized order of takeout fries and washing it down with a medium soda. To save on calories, fat, and sugar, either make your own or look for brands that compare to homemade, such as TruMoo or Nesquik 100 Calorie.

I have a lot of social obligations: birthdays, weddings, and more. I want to join in the celebration without overdoing it. What can I eat?

When these types of occasions occur once in a blue moon, it's easy to say, "Go ahead; enjoy yourself." But every now and then our social calendars seem to overflow with these festive food free-for-alls. There are a few techniques you can use that will allow you to stay on your diet but still enjoy the merriment. The first involves having a little preparty snack. With many of these events, there is so much going on that you find yourself waiting and waiting until the food finally arrives. By then you're so hungry you could eat anything. This is where your snack comes into play. You don't want to eat anything too big, just a little something to prevent your belly from being completely empty once mealtime rolls around. A few examples are:

- A garden salad topped with a handful of nuts
- A few thin slices of low-sodium turkey breast with a few whole grain crackers
- An apple with a tablespoon of peanut butter on top
- A handful of whole grain baked tortilla chips dipped in guacamole

Whatever you choose to eat, wash it down with a glass of skim milk. A recent Australian study demonstrated that skim milk, when compared to a carbohydrate-based beverage such as a juice drink, resulted in study participants eating less food at the following meal. In addition, they stated they had greater feelings of satiety, too.

Once you're at the party, your best course of action depends on the style of the meal—sit down or buffet. For table service, there are a few tricks you can bring out to keep your calorie intake down. Eat the salad, but keep your dressing on the side. Dipping each forkful will cut down on the amount of dressing you use. Plus, researchers out of Penn State have shown that having a first course of a low-energy-dense food, or foods which provide a small amount of calories for a large amount of food, such as a vegetable-filled salad results in fewer calories being consumed in the following meal. If you're eating out, ask your server to serve all sauces and gravies on the side. This lets you control the amount you use and can potentially save you a few hundred calories. With your premeal tricks to curb your appetite, you should be able to enjoy your dinner until you're comfortably full and still keep your weight loss on track.

For buffet-style meals, you'll need to take a slightly different approach. Still take advantage of any low-energy-dense foods like garden salads, fruits, and vegetables to help fill you up. Then, scan the entire buffet. Look for lean meats and baked and steamed items instead of fried foods. Fill your plate using the 50-25-25 rule. Half of your plate should be fruits and veggies, one quarter should be lean meats, and the remaining quarter is for the starch or grain portion of the meal. Plus, limit yourself to one helping of all but the veggies and fruits. No matter what calorie-controlling techniques you use, allow yourself a small serving of dessert if you desire, so you won't feel deprived.

Also, don't underestimate that preparty bar, which is often open long before the food is served at weddings and other parties. This can spell disaster for people watching their weight. Multiple studies have shown that drinking alcohol before a meal leads to a greater number of calories being consumed at that meal. In fact, one study shows that participants took in about 30 percent more calories when they drank. Also, people don't appear to naturally adjust their caloric intake to account for the calories from the drink. Moreover, alcohol not only doesn't force your body to compensate for the extra calories by eating less, it actually stimulates your appetite, causing you to eat more. So if you drink water and then eat a 500-calorie meal, you will have consumed a total of 500 calories, but if you drink a 200-calorie alcoholic beverage before that meal, you will, according to scientific research, still eat all of that 500-calorie meal (and perhaps more), for a total of 700 calories (or more). Stick to carbonated water with a twist or some other calorie-free drinks before your meal and save your alcoholic beverage for once your food arrives.

R_x I eat healthy every day, but I just can't stop my craving for something sweet. What can I eat to satisfy my craving?

Many of us believe healthy eating equals banning favorite foods. Certainly no one would argue that a diet made up entirely of whole grains, lean protein, fresh fruits and veggies, and low-fat dairy foods is healthy. However, for those of us with a sweet tooth, following such a diet 24/7 without exception can be less than enjoyable. In fact, research has shown that dramatic food restrictions can lead to excessive eating, bingeing, and a preoccupation with food—not to mention feelings of guilt for going off your diet. Now suddenly the healthy-eating plan you were so faithful to has turned into a miserable cycle of eating healthy-feeling cravings-bingeing-having guilt.

A better way to look at healthy eating includes not only consuming the foods recommended in this book but also recognizing your ability to include a few less-than-healthy foods once in a while. A few strategically placed splurges or treats built into your eating plan can help prevent overindulgences fueled by deprivation and will keep you on track for a primarily healthy diet.

While it may sound counterintuitive to eat a treat after you've eaten a healthy meal, this is actually the best time. Because of a treat's high sugar content, indulging on an empty stomach will most likely lead to an immediate satisfaction followed very soon after by a giant crash in energy and mood. And, it may leave you hungry as well. The sugar is digested very quickly and gives a quick rush of energy and good feelings, which is nice, but a side effect of that quick digestion and immediate high is a sudden drop. By enjoying your sweet treat *after* a healthy meal, you will find that the protein, fat, and fiber in the meal will help slow the digestion

> ## MAKE IT WORK FOR YOU
>
> A little sweet is fine once in a while, but eating too much can affect more than your weight. Though research into the role diet plays in acne prevention is conflicting, a recent review of several studies showed that diets that include foods with a high sugar content may worsen the development of acne.

Research has shown that too much sugar in the diet may lead to the development of substances that damage the collagen in skin, which leads to dryness, sagging, and wrinkles. Each day, the average American eats about 22 teaspoons of added sugar—sugar actually *added* to foods, not naturally occurring sugars that show up in fruit and dairy products— which equals more than 350 calories. The American Heart Association recommends that women eat no more than 6 teaspoons of added sugar and men no more than 9.

and absorption of the sugars. This means you won't get the instant rush or the miserable low.

Depending on your likes, let yourself have one miniature version of your favorite candy bar with your lunch a few times a week. Even something as simple as adding some chocolate syrup to your milk a couple of times a week may do it for you. Or have a small scoop of ice cream once a week.

If ice cream is your Achilles heel and the multiple gallons and pints of frozen delight call to you nightly from your freezer, you need to know what you're digging into. And don't fool yourself into thinking frozen yogurt is a health food. Here's how the numbers stack up for one half-cup serving of various frozen dairy desserts. (Note that numbers are averages to account for different flavors and brands.)

Ice Cream Comparisons (for ½ cup serving)			
Product	Calories	Total Fat (in grams)	Sugar (in grams)
Super Premium (Ben & Jerry's, etc.)	260	15	23
Regular (Edy's/Dreyer's/Hood, etc.)	160	8	14
Slow Churned/Light	105	3.5	11
Without Added Sugar	110	4	3
Frozen Yogurt	140	3	19
Sherbet	120	1	21
Sorbet (Häagen-Dazs, Ciao Bella, etc.)	100	0.5	20

And if chocolate is your downfall, there are plenty of delicious ways to beat that dreaded craving and still stick to your dieting guns. Believe it or not, there is plenty of chocolate goodness available at a low-calorie price, such as:

- Sugar-free or fat-free chocolate pudding cups
- Chocolate graham crackers
- Hot chocolate made with skim milk—this one even gives you a calcium bonus
- About a teaspoon of Nutella on whole grain toast
- 1 tablespoon of chocolate-covered raisins
- 1 tablespoon of chocolate-covered peanuts
- One or two chocolate candy kisses
- Fresh strawberries or banana slices dipped into 1 tablespoon melted chocolate chips

I know I didn't always specify, but I am now: Stick to whatever the package lists as a serving size for your cocoa treat. Choosing a low-calorie chocolate food won't matter if you eat five servings.

I love the convenience of the healthier frozen meals I often have for lunch or dinner. Is there something as convenient I can have for breakfast?

You can try some of the healthy frozen breakfasts such as Weight Watchers Smart Ones Morning Express and Amy's Kitchen breakfast bowls and scrambles. One big concern with frozen meals, though, is that they tend to be low in calcium and fiber. Still, that's an easy enough problem to fix: simply round out the meal with a cup of yogurt or skim milk and some fresh fruit. This will help get you started on those 1,000 to 1,200 milligrams of calcium you need each day, as well as several vitamins, such as A and C. You can do the same if you choose to have a couple of hardboiled eggs. Two eggs are loaded with enough satisfying protein and nutrients to get you through the morning but only contain 150 calories and 10 grams of fat.

MAKE IT WORK FOR YOU

Getting enough fiber can protect your heart, keep your digestive system running smoothly, and more. Strive to get at least 25 grams of fiber a day. The best sources of fiber are fresh fruits, vegetables, beans, and whole grains. Here's the fiber content, in grams, of a few common foods:

- Black beans, 1 cup—12
- Cooked peas, 1 cup—8.8
- Raspberries, 1 cup—8
- Raisin Bran, 1 cup—6.6
- Whole wheat spaghetti, 1 cup cooked—6.3
- Broccoli, 1 cup cooked—5.1
- Apple, 1 medium with skin—5
- Air-popped popcorn, 3 cups—3.5
- Pistachios, 1 ounce (about 49)—3.4

when to eat what

I'm heading out to an afternoon barbecue. Will there be anything there that can I eat that won't destroy my diet?

Trying to eat healthy at a barbecue certainly presents its challenges. But that's not to say there aren't strategies you can use to make it through the afternoon with your healthy-eating plan still intact. Your battle plan begins before you even arrive. Ask the host or hostess if you can bring something. That way you ensure that you'll have at least one nutritious, figure-friendly dish from which to choose. And make it a nutritional whopper—a brown rice salad packed with chopped veggies and nuts is not only low in fat and calories and filled with vitamins, but also loaded with belly-filling fiber, which will help you say no to some of the less nutritionally beneficial foods. You could also offer to bring an assortment of vegetables that need only be brushed with a scant amount of olive oil, sprinkled with some seasoning, and grilled to perfection. It's a nice change of pace from the usual veggie tray. Veggies that grill well include zucchini, eggplant, and sweet potato slices.

Also, before you get to the food fest, make yourself a little appetizer. I'm not talking mozzarella sticks and chicken wings, I mean something that will take the edge off your appetite so you don't overdo it on the high-cal food and can get through the party subsisting on salad and fruit if need be. Basically, you want a mini meal, such as half a peanut butter or turkey sandwich, a hardboiled egg, and a slice of whole grain toast, or a cup of bean soup with a few whole grain crackers. Wash any of these appetizers down with a glass of skim milk for an extra shot of satisfying protein.

Once you get to the barbeque, you will likely be faced with things like bowls of assorted chips and dips or pepperoni-and-cheese platters. But since you've already had your appetizer at home, you can steer clear of these without those hunger pangs drawing you in. Out of sight, out of mind, so just position yourself away from these nibbles. The main course is often burgers and hot dogs—maybe some sausages or barbecued chicken. Stay away from the hot dogs and sausages. However, a simple, small burger would be a diet-friendly choice. These days they may even have a few veggie burgers on the grill, an even healthier choice. If there's grilled chicken available, grab a breast, peel off the skin, and feel comfortable eating a piece about the size of the palm of your hand.

For a refreshing dessert, try to have some sort of fruit, be it a slice of melon or a colorful salad. Maybe it's the nice weather or the ability to eat outside, but most barbecues seem to have fruit as a dessert option. And just like that, you've enjoyed the barbecue, had a nutritious meal, and your diet is still alive and well.

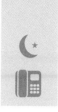

I usually eat dinner around 6:00 P.M., but I sometimes go out with clients for a late dinner around 9:00 P.M. What should I eat to avoid getting too off schedule?

Think of your usual dinnertime as your appetizer time. Enjoy a salad, perhaps some reduced-fat cheese and whole grain crackers, or dried fruit and nuts. These foods will put something in your stomach to help prevent you from binge-ing when you get to the restaurant, where the food most likely isn't as low in calories or fat as your options at home.

At the restaurant, remember you've already had your appetizer, so you can save several hundred calories there. When it comes to ordering your dinner, keep the meal light. Avoid calorie-dense foods such as these:

- Beef
- Other meats such as pork and chicken
- Potatoes
- Creamy soups and sauces
- Pastry
- Fried foods
- Soda
- Alcohol

Instead, choose a dinner that includes:

- Vegetables
- Garden salads (vs. grain-based or meat-filled salads)
- Broth-based soups
- Water
- Fruit
- Seafood (baked, broiled, or poached)

I eat a lot of sugar-free and fat-free treats, but I'm not losing weight. Should I be eating all of these sugar-free goodies?

There's nothing wrong with a sweet little treat, but you may be going about it in all the wrong way. Believe it or not, you may be better off with a non-sugar-free snack. Purdue University researchers found that the addition to one's diet of artificial sweeteners like NutraSweet, Splenda, Sweet'N Low, and stevia found in sugar-free and low-calorie goodies did nothing to help promote weight loss or prevent weight gain. And I have a pretty good idea why: Our brains are sneaky little creatures. They see "sugar free" or even "fat free" on a food label and they relay that message to you as though it said "calorie free" and "eat all you want." But that's just not the case at all. In addition, while many sugar-free foods taste pretty good, they may not taste quite as good as their sugar-filled counterpart. This makes them not quite as satisfying as the real deal. Combine these two issues and you're likely to end up eating far more of the sugar-free goodies than you should. And, as it turns out, many sugar-free or fat-free foods have almost the same amount of calories as their original. (Some even have more.) So, for example, instead of eating maybe two cookies with a bit of real sugar and fat for around 125 calories, you end up eating a dozen or more sugar-free cookies for around 600 calories.

A better idea is to think about what kind of treat you want and eat a small amount of the real thing. Allowing yourself to have a small portion of what you really want versus an artificial substitution allows you to get that pleasure and satisfaction you're looking for without causing overeating. As long as you don't have diabetes or other issues for which you shouldn't eat any sugar, a small amount of real sugar in your diet is ok. Examples of small but satisfying real treats include:

- ¼ cup of a premium ice cream topped with topped with fresh berries or chopped nuts
- 1 ounce of your favorite chocolate

when to eat what

- 1-ounce oatmeal raisin cookie
- 1 slice of pumpkin pie (1/10 of a 10" pie)

Sure, these are small portions, but a little goes a long way. Take small bites and really savor each one to make it last and prolong your enjoyment.

Another way to go in terms of getting a little sweet but not going overboard is the 100-calorie packs. These popular treats have built-in portion control, so you don't need to give it a second thought. You can open one and know that you can eat the whole thing. It's a great feeling, especially when you've been trying to eat less of everything. Go ahead and make your own single-serving sizes of your favorite treats and package them ahead of time. This way when the urge hits, you don't have to mess with that little devil willpower in controlling how much your serve yourself. Go ahead and scoop out a bunch of ½ cup servings of ice cream, and then place each serving in its own self-sealing bag in the freezer so you can simply pull out one bag at a time. The same goes for cookies. Portion out one or two cookies, each in their own bag, and freeze them. The method works especially well with baked goods like cookies because then you don't get that feeling of "I need to eat them all before they go stale." This way, they'll be fresh and calorie controlled for whenever your sweet craving hits.

I try to take a multivitamin to supplement my diet. When's the best time to take it?

Before we start talking about *when* to take vitamins, I want to get the word out that they are not magic bullets. Vitamins are not meant to fix or replace an otherwise unhealthy diet. In addition, if a little is good, more is not always better. There are two types of vitamins: water-soluble and fat-soluble. When it comes to the water-soluble ones, C and all of the Bs, if you eat more than your body needs, your body will just get rid of the excess by excreting it. However, when it comes to fat-soluble vitamins—vitamins A, D, E, and K—that's not the case. If you consume more fat-soluble vitamins than your body needs, they're stashed away in your body. And even though vitamins are nutrients your body needs, continually taking in too much of the fat-soluble ones can lead to toxic levels being stored in your body. So the bottom line is to keep your vitamin intake pretty close to 100 percent of the daily recommended amount.

Now, to answer your question, I look at a daily multivitamin as I look at insurance. You pay into insurance—health, auto, home—but don't live your life planning on using it. A daily multivitamin is like insurance for your health. Even though we try our best to eat healthy, once in a while life puts us in situations where we're trying to lose weight or we may not be able to eat as nutritiously as we'd like. Those are the times the multivitamin kicks in and makes sure our daily nutrient needs are being met. On average, a year's supply of a basic multivitamin is around $15.00 to $20.00. Seems like a pretty good deal to me.

For most vitamin and mineral supplements, it really doesn't matter exactly when, in terms of time of day, you take them. I would, however, recommend taking them at the same time every day. Having a set time for vitamins each day has two benefits: First, it helps you get into a routine, which makes it easier to remember to take them; second, it keeps the supply of nutrients your body is getting steady. Of course, if you are taking supplements that contain additional substances like caffeine or guarana, which may give you problems sleeping if taken at night, then you'd want to take the supplements in the morning.

Some vitamin and mineral supplements work best when they are taken with (or without) certain foods or other supplements. For example, research has shown that iron absorption is increased with foods containing vitamin C, so take an iron supplement before or with a meal containing orange juice, oranges, strawberries, tomatoes, red peppers, or other high-vitamin-C foods. However, calcium blocks the absorption of iron. Therefore, you wouldn't want to take them both at the same meal.

When it comes to supplements, safety can be an issue. You can go almost anywhere and find some sort of vitamins or supplements being sold: at a drugstore, a vitamin store, a grocery store, the mall, a booth at a fair, and so forth. That doesn't mean, however, that you *should* buy them just anywhere and from anyone. Supplements in the United States, let alone other countries, aren't regulated the way food is. You could buy a bottle of brand A one week and it contains 100% supplement A, but buy another brand somewhere else and it may have 50% A and 50% B. But the label on both says the bottle contains supplement A. They aren't necessarily lying, they're just not giving you the whole story. To ensure that you're getting what you think you are, make certain that somewhere on your supplement label it says USP, which stands for United States Pharmacopeia. This is a nongovernment organization that sets standards for vitamins and supplements. In order to include those letters on a supplement, the manufacturers must be meeting the criteria set by this group when it comes to purity, strength, consistency, and quality of the product.

I eat healthy and have always been thin, but ever since I started going through menopause, an extra twenty pounds seems to have befriended me and I can't get rid of it. I'm eating the same foods and amounts as I always have—how can I get rid of this extra weight?

You say extra weight has appeared seemingly overnight though you're eating the same as always, and therein lies the problem: you're eating like a twenty or thirty year old—and maybe you even feel like one—but on the inside, your body has suddenly started acting as if you're a fifty or sixty year old.

It's easy to blame your weight gain on menopause, but in reality, as we age a couple of other things usually occur that are more likely responsible for the weight gain many women begin to experience in their forties and fifties. First, women tend to be less active. If you have kids, they are probably older now; you aren't chasing toddlers anymore. Also, your socializing may revolve more around sedentary activities now, such as going out to dinner, going out for drinks, or going to a movie or show. Younger people tend to choose physical activities for socialization, such as hiking or biking with friends, or playing a game of tennis. You probably don't do much of that anymore. Add to that the fact that part of the aging process involves replacing some of your body's muscle mass with fat. Your muscles burn all the calories you eat, so less muscle means a slower metabolism or fewer calories burned. Can you see now why eating what you always have is suddenly causing weight gain that it didn't before? Plus, there is one thing we *can* blame on hormones. They appear to be responsible for sending the added weight straight to your abdomen instead of spreading it throughout your body. This makes the weight gain even more visible.

Don't throw in the towel yet. None of this means you have to resign yourself to weighing more. On the contrary, it means you just need to be a bit more proactive than before in your strategies to lose weight. There have been multiple studies comparing weight loss in premenopausal versus postmenopausal women. And the good news is that the postmenopausal women were just as successful as the premenopausal women at losing weight. In fact, you could

when to eat what

say they were even more successful because not only did the postmenopausal women lose the same amount of weight, they also made improvements in their blood pressure, triglyceride and glucose levels, and good cholesterol that the premenopausal women did not.

To see the results you are aiming for, you'll need to be pretty committed to your cause. In one of the studies that resulted in weight loss, the women were eating right around 1,300 calories a day. According to the most recent governmental statistic, the average American woman eats about 1,800 calories a day. FYI, those 1,800 calories are an increase from the average intake of forty years ago; in 1971 it was just over 1,500 calories. If you're currently taking in right around 1,800 calories, even getting back down to 1,500 calories a day could potentially add up to a 30-pound loss in a year. If you don't have that much to lose, you can bump your daily calorie intake up a bit.

The two-week menu in the back of the book gives you about 1,600 calories per day, so you can use that as a jumping off point to get you started. This will ensure that you're meeting your nutrient needs. If you don't lose weight following the menus, try cutting back by about 200 calories, or one snack, a day. If you're losing weight but are constantly hungry, you may want to add about 200 calories, or one snack, a day.

The women in the study were also religious about keeping their activity levels up. They walked briskly 10 to 15 miles a week. That may sound like a lot, but really it's just 1½ to 2 miles a day. If you can maintain a pace of 20 minutes per mile, it's just 30 to 40 minutes a day. Keep in mind that the more active you are, the more leeway you have with what you eat.

So, even though it may seem difficult, it's worth it to try to lose your recently gained weight. Gaining an unneeded ten or twenty pounds or more at any time in your life can be harmful to your health. Excessive weight increases your risk of developing high blood pressure and Type 2 diabetes—both of which bring along their own increased risk factors, including stroke, blindness, and kidney damage—and it increases your risk of certain cancers. It's important to think about the whole picture when it comes to the risks and benefits of gaining and losing weight.

I love to order the seasonal fresh fruit plate when I'm out for breakfast, but I find it doesn't hold me very long. What can I add that will help keep me satisfied longer that won't pack a big-calorie punch?

Fruit plates can be a great choice when you go out to breakfast. Fruit is a fantastic source of vitamins, especially C vitamins, and powerful antioxidants like proanthocyanidins, lycopene, and resveratrol that help protect the body from heart disease, cancer, Alzheimer's, and more. Fruits, though not the only source of antioxidants, are certainly one of the best. The clue to knowing how beneficial a food is in terms of antioxidant content can usually be found in its coloring: the darker the better. Deep-blue blueberries, dark-red strawberries or raspberries, bright-orange oranges—all of these are packed with antioxidant power. For this reason, you should try to eat a rainbow of colors each day. Of course, that color needs to be natural. So when you're eating a pink-tinted, strawberry-flavored yogurt with no hint of strawberries, chances are that there aren't any antioxidants to be found in that snack. Do yourself a favor and just buy plain or vanilla yogurt and add your own fresh berries. This will ensure that you're actually getting the nutrients and fruit you need.

You said that fresh fruit by itself leaves you wanting more not long after. Since both fiber and protein take longer to digest than the natural sugar found in fruits, either or both would be great additions to a fruit-based breakfast. But to find the best choices, you often have to read the fine print on your breakfast menu. It's easy to find the Big Bam Slam breakfasts or the Hungry Man Specials on most menus, but you must be diligent and look harder. Look for the little box somewhere near the end of the menu, usually at the bottom of the page that says something like A

> ### MAKE IT WORK FOR YOU
>
> One study has shown that an adequate intake of vitamin C can help maintain younger-appearing skin by minimizing wrinkles as well as the dryness associated with aging. Fruits such as oranges, strawberries, and grapefruit are terrific sources of vitamin C, but so are vegetables including red and green bell peppers and potatoes.

when to eat what

la Carte, or Side Dishes. On that list you'll usually be able to find:

- A bowl of oatmeal
- Whole grain toast
- Cold cereal (look for bran flakes or another whole grain choice that's low in sugar)
- Yogurt
- One egg, any style (poached or boiled eggs usually contain the least fat)

Any of those would make a delicious and satisfying addition to a breakfast of fresh fruit.

MAKE IT WORK FOR YOU

Our bodies are constantly being exposed to conditions or substances that damage them. In the same way a car or metal rusts from extended exposure to the harsh environment, our body shows signs of wear and tear, too. Unprotected exposure to the sun's rays, pollution, smoking, certain chemicals, and even just byproducts of food digestion can all damage our bodies' cells. In fact, much of this damage is responsible for the signs of aging that occur on the outside and inside of our bodies. Eating a variety of antioxidant-rich foods is one of the best actions you can take to minimize this environmental damage.

When I go for my weekly dinner out with my partner, what can I eat from the menu to help me not feel so full after dinner?

Eating out is a wonderful luxury, but many restaurants make it tough to keep your health and weight in mind while doing so. Part of the problem is the excessively large portions that many restaurants serve. Most restaurants serve portions that are anywhere from two and a half to eight times the recommended size, and research has shown that when served food, the majority of people are more likely to eat all that's in front of them instead of leaving some or bringing some home. So it's time to buck the trend. There's nothing wrong with bringing half your meal home. Look at it as a readymade lunch for the next day. The best way to do this is to ask your server to wrap half up as soon as he or she brings your plate. This will solve any problems with willpower you may have once you dig in.

In addition, usually when you go out to eat, you've barely cracked open the menu and you have food already—chips and salsa, breadsticks, warm rolls and butter, focaccia and olive oil. It doesn't matter what form it comes in, because it all boils down to one thing: extra calories that you don't need. When you arrive, kindly ask your server not to bring it. Problem solved.

Another huge calorie and discomfort saver—skip the appetizer. Even if you share an appetizer with your partner, you could both end up eating anywhere from about 300 to 700 extra calories before your dinner even arrives. If you feel you really need something before your meal arrives, try a veggie-filled salad or a broth-based soup instead. Research has shown that both of these types of foods can result in fewer calories being consumed in the meal that follows.

At the end of the meal, when it comes to something sweet, my first suggestion is to share with your partner, and maybe even leave some on the plate to bring home for another night. Many of these restaurant desserts can easily contain 700, 800, or 900 calories (or more!). Stick to the simple desserts like cookies or ice cream. Many restaurants, like PF Chang's and Carrabba's Italian Grill, are now offering mini desserts, which are a great way to get a sweet-treat finale without needing to loosen your belt.

when to eat *what*

I've never been a coffee drinker, but I'm addicted to cola. I know regular soda has a lot of empty calories so I drink diet. With no calories, it's just as good for me as water, right?

The jury is still out on that. There's a lot of research showing that the artificial sweeteners may hinder weight loss because they interfere with your body's ability to regulate appetite. Basically, your body becomes confused when you eat something sweet but don't get any calories or energy from it. But, regardless of the reason why, there's more interesting research out there that may very well have you trading in that can of diet soda for a bottle of water.

Researchers at the Stanford Prevention Research Center looked at the difference between drinking water and calorie-free sweet drinks such as diet soda, diet juices, diet sweetened teas, and diet lemonades and other fruity drinks. All of the participants were following some sort of diet to lose weight. Not surprisingly, the mere act of drinking water regularly prompted a five-pound weight loss per year. When participants replaced their sugary drinks with water, they lost even more weight. The exact amount was dependent on how many sugary drinks they drank and how many they replaced with water. But the real kicker here was that when the drinkers replaced sugary drinks with diet drinks, they only lost about three and a half pounds in the year compared to greater than five by replacing the caloric sugar-filled drinks with water.

In your situation, if you feel that you need the caffeine from the diet cola, perhaps limiting yourself to one a day at the time you need it most would be the most beneficial. Then drink water the remainder of the day.

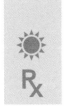

It's only 30 minutes before I'm normally going to have lunch, but I'm so hungry I'm not feeling well. What should I eat?

You want something that's going to start quelling that hunger—and sick feelings—right away. Simple carbohydrates are the answer. Our bodies digest them quickly, which makes them perfect for these kinds of situations. You'll be eating soon, so you don't need to worry about something with staying power like protein or fiber. Go for fruit and/or some simple grains. Try one of the following:

- A small glass of 100% fruit juice and a piece of toast
- A few crackers and grapes
- A couple of whole wheat mini pitas with all-fruit spread
- Dried fruit and ready-to-eat whole grain cereal such as Cheerios or Kix

Knowing how to prevent these feelings of starvation in the future can be helpful, too. I suspect that when this happens, breakfast was hours ago. If you think of your body as a car and food as the gas that fuels it, those feelings of starvation are like your car coasting in on fumes to the gas station. You're lucky you made it as far as you did. Prevent this type of hunger from happening in the first place by going no longer than 3 or 4 hours without eating and planning a healthy between-meals snack if necessary. The ideas mentioned in this section make great snacks, and the two-week menu in the back of the book is also full of snack ideas.

If you want fruit but worry about carrying it around, try dried fruits. They're a great way to get the disease-fighting nutrients and anti-oxidants found in fruit without possible spills, damage, or spoilage in a lunch bag or backpack. Broaden your dried-fruit horizons beyond raisins and Craisins and try dried blueberries, raspberries, strawberries, peaches, pineapples, apples, apricots, and more. One word of warning: If you're looking to try some dried bananas, watch out for banana chips. Often these are fried, which means they contain a lot more calories and fat than a dried fruit.

when to eat what

I know how important eating breakfast is to losing weight, but so many breakfast foods are dairy foods or include them. I'm lactose intolerant. What can I eat for breakfast that won't irritate my digestive system?

It's been estimated that roughly 50 million adults in the United States have lactose intolerance to some extent. Lactose intolerance is when the body cannot properly digest the sugars found in milk and other dairy products. Symptoms range from mild discomfort to painful cramping, gas, diarrhea, and more. Unfortunately, people suffering from this condition end up avoiding dairy products; this may help prevent their symptoms but it also may keep them from attaining adequate levels of certain nutrients found largely in dairy foods. Luckily, there are other options.

There are also products available to help people with lactose concerns. You can buy lactase supplements in most drug and grocery stores—lactase is the enzyme required to digest the milk sugar lactose. These supplements are not drugs; they are enzymes the body makes. It's just that in people with lactose intolerance, for whatever reason, this enzyme isn't doing its job. The Lactaid company also makes a variety of milks, cheeses, ice creams, and more that don't contain lactose. So, between yogurt, smaller portions, lactose-reduced foods and drinks, and lactase supplements, there should be nothing stopping you from starting your day with a healthy, balanced, dairy-delightful breakfast.

MAKE IT WORK FOR YOU

In many people, lactose digestion is only a problem when large quantities of dairy products are eaten without other foods. To prevent this while still enjoying dairy foods, simply spread your intake of dairy foods out more throughout the day so you can have smaller servings. Also, always include other foods with your dairy. So instead of drinking a big glass of milk, have ½ cup of milk on a bowl of whole grain cereal or have a small glass of milk with a meal. In addition, most people with lactose intolerance have no problems digesting yogurt, which is a great breakfast staple.

I'm going out for drinks with friends later but don't want to get tipsy. Is there anything I can eat before we order our drinks?

In a word, anything. Just getting something in your stomach will help you not get drunk so quickly. Researchers have found that when you eat a meal about an hour or so before drinking, your blood alcohol level will only be 64 percent of someone who fasted before drinking, assuming you each drank the same amount. That's a big difference. Researchers believe that the presence of food in the stomach slows the speed at which the contents of the stomach—the food and alcohol—empty into the intestines, where they are absorbed into the blood stream. But there's more. Eating before drinking also left the drinkers feeling less drunk. Compared to those who were fasting, they actually metabolized the alcohol much quicker, about two hours faster, and the alcohol left their bloodstream much faster—about 35 to 50 percent faster. Not only does eating before drinking get you less drunk, it appears as though it may help you sober up faster, too.

So now that you understand why it's so important to eat, the question becomes what should you eat. An initial study showed that eating a mixed meal of carbohydrate, fat, and protein helps blood alcohol levels return to normal 25 percent faster than when the same amount of alcohol is consumed on an empty stomach. Researchers then took it one step further. They did the same basic study, except this time, instead of one meal, the participants ate one of three meals. One was a high-fat meal, one was a high-protein meal, and the third was a high-carbohydrate meal. It turned out that the type of meal made no difference, but alcohol was

when to eat what

eliminated from the body 45 percent faster than in those who had no meal. Subsequent studies have been completed with similar results.

Since the type of food doesn't seem to matter, I'd recommend a low-fat meal that includes lean protein. You don't need the extra calories a high-fat meal would provide, and the protein will help keep you feeling fuller longer, which may make saying no to high-calorie bar snacks easier. A large salad topped with grilled chicken, a hardboiled egg, or drained water-packed tuna would be a good predrinking meal. A simpler meal could be a tuna or egg salad sandwich on whole wheat bread along with a piece of fruit.

I've recently lost a lot of weight on one of those plans in which they provide the food and the shakes. I'm afraid I'll put it all back on once I go back to real food. What and when should I eat to prevent that?

Oftentimes, people find weight maintenance harder than weight loss, so I can understand your fears. Remember that this is not an all-or-nothing situation. You don't need to make an all-at-once switch from the prepackaged diet foods to food you prepare yourself. In fact, a study on weight loss showed that after the initial weight loss phase of prepackaged diets like this, continuing to eat one prepackaged diet meal replacement a day for up to a couple of years after you reintroduce regular food was beneficial in keeping the lost weight off and resulted in a slightly greater weight loss. So just start with one meal at a time and make the switch gradually.

The morning is often when our willpower is at its peak. We've just woken up, refreshed and ready to start the day. That and the fact that breakfast foods tend to be the easiest to prepare and contain many ingredients that are naturally

MAKE IT WORK FOR YOU

Being aware of what constitutes a serving of various foods is crucial when it comes to keeping portion sizes under control. Here are a few examples of what equals one serving from each of the food groups.

- Dairy group: 8 ounces milk or yogurt, 1 to 1½ ounces cheese

- Fruit group: 1 medium piece, ½ cup sliced or small fruits, 2 tablespoons dried, ½ cup 100% fruit juice

- Vegetable group: ½ cup cooked vegetables, 1 cup raw or leafy vegetables

- Grain group: 1 slice bread, ½ cup cooked cereal (e.g., oatmeal), 1 cup dry cereal, ½ cup cooked pasta, ½ cup cooked rice, ½ an English muffin or hamburger bun

- Protein group: 1 tablespoons peanut butter, 1 large egg, 3 ounces lean meat, 1 ounce nuts

when to eat what

healthy makes breakfast the ideal meal with which to start your transition to "real" food. One of the hardest parts of this type of change is keeping portion sizes in check. It will be most helpful, at least at first, to weigh and measure foods to ensure you're not eyeballing too large a serving.

While the measuring and weighing may seem like a pain, it's the most accurate way of knowing exactly what you're eating and making sure that you're not eating more than you should.

Next, look at the prepackaged meals you ate. What was in them? What wasn't? Use them as a guide for creating your own healthy, homemade versions. Ever have an egg sandwich for breakfast? Create one yourself with one egg and some multigrain bread or a multigrain English muffin. Pair it with some fruit and skim milk and you've made a healthy breakfast. Once you're feeling more comfortable preparing one meal a day from scratch, move on to another. It doesn't even have to be a full meal. Perhaps creating some healthy snacks might seem a bit less daunting. If your diet plan included snacks, look at some of the labels to get a rough idea of how many calories they were, along with the amount of protein, fiber, and sugar they contained. You can then compare them to items from the grocery store to figure out how foods without labels, such as fresh fruits and vegetables, can fit into your plan. You might also want to try using an online calorie calculator such as *www.caloriecount.com*. It may be a lot of work in the beginning, but it'll all pay off in the end when you're eating food you've made from scratch and keeping off that weight.

My doctor has recommended a calcium supplement. When is the best time to take it?

It depends on what type you're taking. There are two types of calcium supplements: calcium carbonate, such as Caltrate or Tums; and calcium citrate, such as Citracal. If you're taking calcium carbonate, you want to be sure to take it with meals because it needs the stomach acids produced when you eat to maximize absorption. If you're taking calcium citrate, you can take it either with or without meals, whatever works for you. The recommended daily intake for calcium for adults is 1,000 to 1,200 milligrams. Most supplement tablets contain 500 to 600 milligrams. That means you'll most likely be taking 2 tablets if you're taking a calcium supplement. Calcium absorption is best when you take in about 500 milligrams or less at a time. So if you are taking two tablets, just split the dose and take them at two different times per day.

In addition, iron interferes with the absorption of calcium, so if you're taking calcium and a multivitamin or other supplement which contains iron, here's one way you could do it. First, take the calcium at breakfast and lunch. Then, take the multivitamin with iron with a dinner that contains some vitamin C-rich foods. (Also see "I try to take a multivitamin to supplement my diet. When's the best time to take it?" for more info.)

MAKE IT WORK FOR YOU

You know that calcium builds strong bones, but you may not know that vitamin D is needed to help calcium be absorbed and used properly. Two recent studies showed that women who consumed the recommended daily amount of each actually gained less weight over several years than those who didn't. Most, if not all, calcium-rich foods contain or are fortified with vitamin D. If you're using a supplement, just make sure you're getting 400IU of vitamin D along with your calcium.

when to eat what

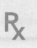

R_x I'm pregnant and am always craving something. What should I eat when a craving hits?

When it comes to cravings during pregnancy, it is especially important to consider what you've already eaten on that particular day. Take a look at the food groups from which you have *not* met your daily needs yet and try to choose snacks from those groups. Of course, there are times when all thoughts of nutrition fly out the window and you want what you want. During those times, check out these ideas, which are based on the food groups and the kinds of cravings they satisfy, to help you make the right decision.

- **Grain:** Whole grain crackers (crunchy, salty); whole grain toast (comforting); air-popped or light microwave popcorn (crunchy); whole grain cereal (comforting, crunchy); whole grain pretzels (crunchy, salty)
- **Dairy:** Chocolate milk made with skim or 1% milk (comforting, chocolate); low-fat yogurt (creamy, sweet); reduced-fat cheese (creamy, comforting); pudding made with low-fat milk or a fat-free pudding cup (sweet, creamy)
- **Vegetables:** Salsa (spicy, salty); baby carrots/celery sticks (crunchy); small baked potato (warm, comforting); baked sweet potato fries (warm, comforting, sweet)
- **Fruit:** Raisins, Craisins, dried blueberries, or other dried fruit (sweet, chewy); frozen whole-fruit/sorbet bar (frozen, sweet); fresh fruit (crunchy, sweet, juicy)
- **Protein:** Peanut butter (creamy, sweet, comforting); hummus (salty, creamy); nuts (crunchy, salty); hardboiled egg (warm, comforting); edamame (crunchy)

While it is important to eat nutritiously and ensure you're getting enough calories to support you and the pregnancy, you don't want to take the old adage about eating for two too much to heart. In actuality, the calorie recommendations for pregnancy are only 300 more per day than your usual calorie needs when you're not pregnant. That means you have far less wiggle room for indiscriminant calories, so make sure as much as possible that every calorie you eat is nutrient packed rather than just full of sugar, fat, and salt.

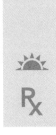

I love the protein boost and appetite-curbing power of eggs in the morning, but what is the best way to prepare them to get the biggest dietary bang for my buck?

You're certainly on the right track with eggs; they are a great culinary blank canvas that you can use to create all kinds of nutritious meals. And even though eggs have gotten a bad rap, they are extremely nutritious. In fact, they are an excellent source of the amino acid leucine, which has been shown in studies to play a role in controlling hunger—a key factor when you're trying to lose weight.

In this day and age of super-nonstick pans, you can pretty much prepare an egg with any method and have it be figure friendly. That being said, those preparations that traditionally require no additional fat whatsoever—hardboiled, soft boiled, and poached—are probably the best choices since you still may need to add some fat to a nonstick pan. These preparations are terrific when paired with whole grain toast for some fiber, B vitamins, and whole grains.

But this doesn't mean that other types of eggs are out of the question. Egg scrambles and omelets are both good options when you want to add more to a simple egg breakfast. For example, for a calcium boost, you can add low-fat cheese. But if you really want a nutritional and weight-watching knockout, adding veggies is the way to go. Most have 25 or fewer calories per ½ cup but are full of fiber and water. All that adds up to a food that fills you up without filling you out. You could realistically add

when to eat what

2 cups of diced vegetables to two eggs to create a hearty, nutritious breakfast for only 250 calories and 10 grams of fat. In fact, this breakfast is so low in calories, you will probably want to add some fruit or whole grain toast to it as well.

Another way to boost protein without adding additional fat is to add more egg whites. Each adds only 17 calories, and they scramble up perfectly with whole eggs.

A word of advice, though. I often hear people talk about, and see on menus, egg-white omelets. In my opinion, eating only the whites is a bit extreme, and it can even lead to missed-out nutritional opportunities. Even when you cook up four egg whites in an omelet, you're still eating less than 80 calories for breakfast. This is not enough to be beneficial to weight loss or to get you through to the next hour, let alone lunch.

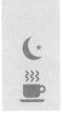

Most weeknights I tend to fall asleep on the couch by 8:00. Is there anything that I can do to stay awake a bit longer?

My first thought, if we're strictly talking food here, is that perhaps you're eating a bit too many carbs in the afternoon: lots of breads, pastas, crackers, chips, pretzels, French fries, pastries, and other carbohydrate-dense foods. These foods are known to be very calming, which would explain why you're so tired at night. The same can apply to dairy products. In the afternoon, make sure you have a good balance of some carbohydrates, a bit of dairy, and some protein to avoid overdosing on any of it, which may force you into an unplanned early slumber.

Another consideration is to eat enough food at lunch and during the afternoon to make sure you're getting the energy your body needs; otherwise, you will feel tired. Aim for around 400 calories from your lunch and then another 150 to 200 from an afternoon snack each day, choosing foods that allow these calories to be a mixture of protein, fat, and carbohydrates. That means selecting lean proteins such as beans, skinless chicken, seafood, or lean beef; along with whole grains like 100% whole grain bread, whole grain crackers, or other whole grain types of bread; fruits; vegetables; low-fat dairy such as skim or 1% milk, nonfat yogurt, or reduced-fat cheese; and healthy fats like salad dressing made from canola or olive oil, avocados, or other fats such as reduced-fat sandwich spreads or mayonnaise or soft tub margarine.

when to eat what

I love to sleep in on the weekends. How should I alter my eating from my weekday routine to fit a different morning schedule?

Lounging in bed a bit longer than usual is certainly a nice treat, but don't let it turn you into a lazy eater. After all, it's never too late to start your day in a healthy way. The best idea for you is to turn your usual meal-snack-meal-snack morning through early afternoon routine into a meal-snack-snack routine. Enjoy a hearty brunch in place of breakfast and lunch (as long as it's not at the local all-you-can-eat diner!), and then have a small snack shortly after your usual lunchtime and another at your usual afternoon snack time.

Approximately 300 to 400 calories is usually a decent-sized breakfast for the average person, so for a brunch, since you're essentially combining two meals but don't want to go overboard, I'd aim for around 500 or 600 calories. The benefit of brunch is that it usually contains the same whole grain, fruit, and low-fat dairy options found in breakfast but is also more conducive to meats and vegetables. A great veggie-and-ham-filled frittata can be accompanied by a slice of whole grain French toast filled with fruit and topped with yogurt. This will allow you to extend the pleasure of a relaxing morning into the day without overindulging and feeling the consequences in your waistline and your mood.

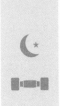

I like to exercise after work, but often find myself dragging by the end of the workout. How can I get the energy I need to exercise without feeling weighed down?

Exercising after work is a great way to get healthy, and your best bet is to leave your workplace and head right for the health club or go straight for your walk or jog. Otherwise, if you go home first, you may decide to flip through the mail, sit down a minute, and then just like that your exercise plans are out the window. Still, when you jump right into your exercise plan after work, you're expecting that lunch you had hours ago not only to last you until dinnertime but also to get you through a workout too. Unfortunately, there's only so far a few hundred calories can go.

When you plan to work out before dinner, bump your afternoon snack up to a mini meal that includes some fiber and protein, and eat it halfway between your lunch and your workout to ensure that your snack is digested and absorbed for your body to use. Because carbohydrates are your body's main energy source, you also want to be sure they play a role in your snack selection. Easy ideas include:

- Mini whole wheat pitas with hummus
- Reduced-fat cheese cubes and whole grain crackers
- An apple with peanut butter
- Nonfat plain or vanilla yogurt with nuts and fruit

And don't forget to hydrate. If you don't tend to drink much at work, try to drink a couple of cups of water in the hour or so prior to your workout. You can also bring a cooler or reusable bottle filled with water to sip on as you exercise.

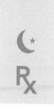

I blew it. By 4:30 I'd eaten all the calories I need in a day. What can I eat for dinner or if I get hungry in the evening that won't make me gain weight?

The good news is that it's highly unlikely that any healthy dinner you eat will make you gain weight, as long as this isn't happening on a daily basis. To gain one pound on any given day, you need to eat about 3,500 calories beyond your body's day-to-day needs. Say you need 1,800 calories a day and by 4:30 they're all used up. You would have to eat the equivalent of roughly 6½ Big Macs that evening to gain one pound. That's a lot of food! But, if you do that math further, you can see that if you blow all of your calories before dinner on a daily basis, having a dinner the size of just one Big Mac every day would increase your weight by a pound in just one week. And none of this is to say you don't want to make a healthy dinner selection.

In this situation, you want to include protein in your final meal of the day to ensure that the fullness and satisfaction you feel after you eat will last through the evening. Otherwise, you may be looking for snacks later on. Vegetables also make a great choice because they're full of water and fiber to help fill you up but are extremely low in calories. A few ideas are:

- Bean chili with a salad
- Bean-and-veggie-filled wrap
- Grilled fish or skinless chicken with steamed vegetables
- A large garden salad topped with drained water-packed tuna or a hardboiled egg

You also need to look at how this happened and figure out what can be done to prevent it in the future. Was it just one of those days when you had a big business lunch, it was someone's birthday, and other rare situations popped up all at the same time? If so, then you just need to finish the day and get on with the next. However, if this happens on a regular basis because you're feeling hungry during the day and can't stop munching, then it may be time to change your daily eating routine a bit.

Perhaps you're not eating enough protein or fiber to provide lasting fullness. In addition, maybe you're eating too many simple carbohydrates and artificially sweetened carbs that speed through your body and continually leave you wanting more. Or maybe you're simply eating large portions of high-calorie, high-fat foods. Identify the problem, make a plan to correct it, and soon you'll be able to regain control of your calorie intake over the course of the day.

when to eat *what*

What can I stash in my emergency snack pack in the car for when I get stuck somewhere or I'm out longer than I had planned?

An emergency stash is a great idea. Life is full of unexpected turns, and you never know when a meeting or shopping trip may take longer than planned or an overwhelming hunger may hit. When you're that hungry, you may be tempted to swing into the closest drive-through restaurant or grab a quick candy bar or bag of chips from the checkout line or a gas station. At these times, having an emergency stash at an arm's length can keep you from derailing your diet.

But what to store in your stash? Often, quenching your thirst can help quell your hunger. Before you head out for the day, fill an insulated bottle with water so you can stay hydrated while on the go. For a more flavorful thirst quencher, you could also try a box of ultra-high-temperature pasteurized milk. If you haven't seen them, look in the coffee, baby food, or health food aisle of your grocery store. They look like little juice boxes but contain milk that is stable to be stored at room temperature. You can keep one or both by your keys and grab them on the way out the door.

Once your thirst is quenched, you'll be ready to sink your teeth into something. Car-stable snacks include 1-ounce packages of nuts, boxes of raisins, baggies of dried fruits, whole grain crackers, fruit-and-grain bars, and low-sugar, low-fat granola bars.

MAKE IT WORK FOR YOU

Granola sounds like it should be healthy, but often it's not. To find truly healthy granola and granola bars, be prepared to do a bit of sleuthing to make sure you're not getting more than you bargained for. Many granolas are filled with fat and sugar, and with their chocolate coatings and candy fillings, many granola bars are no better than a candy bar. Look for ones containing oats and other whole grains, and ingredients you could actually find in your kitchen instead of a laboratory. Also, per bar, try to keep calories around 100 calories, fat under 3 grams, and sugar under 7 grams.

I love to chew gum during the day; it keeps me from munching on other things. Is there anything wrong with popping gum in my mouth as a substitute for eating?

If chewing on gum is keeping you from munching on more calorie-dense foods, then no, there's nothing wrong with it. Researchers recently found that study participants who chewed gum snacked less between lunch and dinner than those who didn't chew gum. The chewers chewed sugarless gum for about 15 minutes out of each hour and consumed about 40 calories less than the non-chewers. That may not sound like much, but 40 calories here and there a couple of times a day adds up. Plus, when it comes to successful weight loss, it's often much easier to maintain many smaller changes that add up than to stick to one or two big changes.

Note that this study involved sugarless gum. A piece of gum with sugar has about 25 calories. That may not sound like a lot, but just like the 40 calories you could potentially save, it adds up. Let's say you chew a fresh piece of gum with sugar every hour during an eight-hour workday. Multiply 25 calories by eight pieces of gum and you've consumed 200 calories.

Chewing gum between meals is all well and good, but be sure you're not chewing gum in place of meals in hopes of saving a few extra calories. You'll not only miss out on valuable nutrients, but you'll also put yourself through a calorie deprivation that will most likely result in overeating later in the day and into the night. In addition, because gum stimulates saliva production, you may not feel the need or desire to drink as much as your body requires, so you may risk becoming dehydrated. To counteract this, drink a glass of water each time you're getting ready to pop a stick of gum into your mouth to ensure that you're getting enough fluids.

MAKE IT WORK FOR YOU

Chewing gum does more than help you not munch as much. British researchers found that chewing gum can help you out mentally as well as physically. When chewing gum, study participants reported being in a better mood. They were also more alert and had a better attention span and reaction time. So when you need a little pick-me-up, pop in a stick of your favorite gum.

when to eat what

In the past, I've followed those diets where you just drink a shake for breakfast and lunch. It was really convenient to simply drink something in the morning and not worry about food, so now I usually have some OJ and coffee and I'm out the door. With such a little breakfast, you'd think I'd be losing weight, but I'm not. What can I drink for breakfast to help me lose weight?

You're not going to like my answer. If you're trying to lose weight, a liquid diet just won't cut it. Numerous studies have been conducted on the subject and they all produce the same results: liquid calories simply do not produce the same lasting feelings of fullness that solid calories do. Certainly, having something to drink before your meal will help you eat fewer calories, and liquids do fill your stomach a bit, but the fullness doesn't last. Your hunger, which was never really satisfied in the first place, comes back, and you'll probably reach for a snack—most likely a pretty large one since your body feels like it missed a meal. So at 10:30 or so, you've had roughly 250 calories from your juice and coffee with a little cream and sugar plus, say, 400 more from your snack. But . . . if you just eat a simple breakfast—say 350 calories plus a small snack, say 100 calories—you'll get through to lunch on about 200 calories less than you will if you keep going on your current liquid diet. The 200 or so calories you'll save daily in this manner by eating a healthy breakfast can add up to a weight loss of about half a pound a week.

Remember, breakfast doesn't have to be anything fancy or elaborate. Simple foods usually make the easiest and healthiest breakfasts. Keep your pantry stocked with some basic breakfast foods and you should have no problem creating a simple breakfast that will help that weight start to drop. Basic breakfast staples include:

- Eggs, fresh and hardboiled
- Whole grain bread, English muffins, pitas, and wraps
- Peanut butter and assorted nuts

- Whole grain ready-to-eat cereals such as Cheerios, Life, Fiber One, and Raisin Bran, to name a few
- Oatmeal—in bulk and instant plain packets
- Skim or 1% milk
- Low-fat and nonfat yogurts—plain or vanilla and flavored
- Fruit—fresh, dried, and juice-packed canned

when to eat what

I usually only have cereal for breakfast, but I don't seem to be losing weight. What am I doing wrong?

Cereal is often recommended as a healthy way to start the morning. But opening just any old box and pouring a big bowlful may not be the best choice. First, you need to get your portion size under control. For most cereals, 1 cup is considered one serving. However, when many of us start pouring our cereal into the bowl we end up with much more, probably about 2 cups, if not more. If this sounds familiar, measure out 1 cup of cereal into a bowl a few times, until you can eyeball what a cup is. Then use that same bowl every time you have cereal to help ensure you're not being a bit too heavy-handed in the pouring department.

Next, look at the type of cereal you're crunching. I usually recommend whole grain cereal, but these days that can lead to confusion, because many bright boxes of sugar-coated cereal boast whole grains. These aren't the kinds of cereal you should be eating regularly, at least not if you're waiting for the numbers on your bathroom scale to come down. Look for a cereal with a whole grain—such as wheat, oats, corn, or brown rice—as the first ingredient and try to find one with 6 or fewer grams of sugar per serving. In addition, when it comes to wheat, look for whole wheat or 100 percent whole wheat to ensure you're getting a whole grain vs. processed wheat or white flour.

Think the bowl size and the specific types of cereal you're eating don't really make a big difference? Consider this: 1 cup of Cheerios or Kix contains between 80 and 100 calories and 1 to 2 grams of sugar. On the other hand, 2 cups of Froot Loops or Cocoa Pebbles has between 240 and 320 calories and 25 to 30 grams of sugar. Which one do you think would be the better choice if you're trying to lose weight?

MAKE IT WORK FOR YOU

The benefits of breakfast have long been touted. It's been shown to lower one's risk of a variety of diseases ranging from diabetes to cardiovascular problems. We've also seen that starting every day with breakfast helps prevent overeating later in the day. It's no wonder that researchers at Harvard School of Public Health found that eating breakfast appeared to be beneficial in preventing weight gain.

R$_X$ I'm a vegetarian. What can I eat for lunch and dinner that will still fill me up and help me lose weight?

Losing weight while following a vegetarian lifestyle isn't necessarily a guarantee, but it certainly is possible. A study from the University of Pittsburgh found that participants on a weight-loss diet who were lacto-ovo vegetarians (they drank milk and ate dairy products and eggs) lost no more or less weight than those following the same type of diet that included meat. That's the bad news. The good news is they all lost weight. At first glance, one would think losing weight would be natural when you're eating like a vegetarian, because your diet contains none of that high-fat red meat, fatty chicken skin, bacon, or hot dogs. But you may still be eating plenty of foods that are not low in fat and calories: French fries, pastries, candy, soda, and so forth. As well, someone on a vegetarian weight-loss diet may still eat portions of pasta, rice, or even beans that are too large. Just like omnivorous dieters, those following a vegetarian diet must make wise choices when trying to lose weight.

First, although you don't mention breakfast, note that any of the healthy breakfast ideas mentioned throughout this book will work for you. However, when you get to lunch and dinner, decisions can get a bit tougher. Later in the book you'll find a section on how to modify the meal plan if you're a vegetarian. You can refer to it to get you started and give you several weight control-friendly ideas. When you're ready to expand on that menu, here are some guidelines to help. You want to make sure you eat enough protein for a satisfying, low-calorie meal, but you don't want to simply dump cheese or spread peanut butter on everything.

Years ago, you needed to go to a health food store to buy your food if you weren't eating meat. Now most supermarkets carry an assortment of soy-based meat replacements. It's easy to find a variety of veggie burgers or soy-and-vegetable-based hamburger alternatives, such as Gardenburgers, Boca burgers, and products from Morningstar Farms. Some are designed to give you that real burger sensation, while others are filled with more vegetables or have an Italian or Latin taste. Feel like having a hot dog but know the fat and sodium (not to

when to eat what

mention the meat) make them a no-no? Try a soy dog, like Yves. They're low in fat, calories, sodium, and no meat!

You can also try soy crumbles and ground beef–like proteins; these are made by companies such as Morningstar Farms, Boca, Lightlife, and Gardenburger. Basically, they have a consistency similar to ground beef, but they are made from something called texturized vegetable protein (TVP). These are a great substitute in any dish in which you would use ground beef, such as sloppy joes, lasagna, casseroles, spaghetti sauce, meatballs, and meatloaf. These products are low in calories and sodium, with little to no fat. They are really a fantastic addition to the vegetarian marketplace to allow greater variety and better nutrition.

Another soy-based protein source is tofu. The wonderful thing about tofu is that it doesn't really have much flavor, so it will take on whatever spices and flavors you cook it with. Tofu can be used in place of meat in a stir-fry, sweet-and-sour dish, chili, casserole, and much more. It can also be blended into smoothies and desserts to add a low-fat, nutrient-filled, protein punch to those items. Tofu varieties include regular and silken, and within those two categories there are several different textures from soft to extra firm. Different styles work better in different dishes, so check out some recipes to learn what you can do with the different types, and then experiment a bit.

To round out the soy-based options in vegetarian cooking, there's edamame (whole soybeans). Packages of edamame (in and out of their pods) are most often found in the frozen foods aisle at the grocery store and have a number of delicious uses. Those in the pods make a great snack—just boil them about 5 minutes and you're good to go with or without a little sprinkle of kosher salt. The preshelled ones make a great addition to salads, pasta salads, bean salads, and more.

You can also try protein-packed beans, such as black, white, red, navy, and kidney, which are a perfect choice for a high-protein, meatless meal. With so many varieties available, you could have a different kind of bean every day and still have some to spare. Beans make a great basis for meatless chilis, tacos, wraps, quesadillas, and more. Plus, in addition to the protein, they're full of fiber to give you twice the filling power. If you find that you experience unpleasant side effects from beans, try taking a supplement like Beano. Beano contains an enzyme, not a drug, which helps your body break down what it can't. Simply take it before a meal that contains beans, and it will be ready to start doing its job as soon as the food gets in there.

And, of course, there's always nuts and nut butters. A simple old-fashioned peanut butter and banana sandwich once in a while makes a great lunch. Nuts are a perfect between-meal snack that can also be used in cooking to add variety, flavor, nutrition, and protein to a meal. For instance, peanut butter makes a delicious sauce for a Thai-inspired veggie-filled stir-fry.

If you replace the meat in your diet with any variety of these healthy foods while you follow a low-fat diet, weight loss shouldn't be a problem. In fact, the majority of these meat alternatives are much lower in calories and fat than their animal-based counterparts, so as long as you watch your intake of the extras—the fried foods, pastries, candy, chips, and so on—following a low-fat vegetarian diet should be a piece of cake.

I like to work out in the evening. When and what should I eat for dinner so I'm not starving halfway through my workout?

With an after-dinner workout, you might be better off splitting your dinner into two smaller meals. Numerous studies have shown that carbohydrates eaten about an hour before you work out allow you to exercise longer before you fatigue, so you get a better workout. Maximizing your performance while working out can improve weight loss.

You'll want to replace some of the carbohydrates you used up during your workout. Just as important, you'll want to be sure you eat enough protein to keep you satisfied through the night. Taking those two concerns into consideration, it may be best to eat the starchy/carb portion of your dinner before you work out along with a glass of skim or 1% milk to get some hydration. After you finish exercising, add in the protein and vegetable part of your evening meal. Here are suggestions for divided dinners; for more dinner ideas you can divide, check out the menu and recipes at the end of the book:

MAKE IT WORK FOR YOU

Stretching before you work out is important no matter what time of day you exercise. Chances are, the muscles you'll be using while exercising are different from those you used the rest of the day. Therefore, you will need a good warm-up. Nothing can be more frustrating and impede a good workout routine more than an injury that could have been prevented with a few minutes of some simple stretching.

Meal Suggestions	
Preworkout Meal	**Postworkout Meal**
Baked potato, fruit salad, milk	Grilled chicken breast, steamed green beans
Spaghetti with marinara sauce, seedless grapes, milk	Meatballs, garden salad
Baked beans, pineapple, milk	Green salad (edamame, green beans)
Macaroni and cheese, melon	Three-bean salad

I'm usually half asleep when I get ready for work in the morning. Sometimes I forget to eat breakfast. Then I end up munching on whatever junk I can find at work until my next meal. What can I eat instead of the junk food at work?

I have a couple of suggestions for you. First, is it possible to set your alarm a few minutes earlier so you have time to fully waken before you head out the door? Second, plan your breakfast the night before. Make breakfast virtually impossible to miss.

Each evening, go ahead and get out a bowl and spoon and a glass. You could even put the cereal box right out on the counter. Have a banana set out or another piece of fruit in the fridge by the milk carton. When you wake up in the morning, breakfast will take no time or thought at all to prepare. A few more prep-ahead ideas include:

- **For yogurt and fruit:** Place a spoon on top of your coffee cup or car keys. Prewash and cut strawberries in a bowl. Place this next to the yogurt, front and center in the fridge.
- **Toast:** Put a loaf of bread, knife, and plate on the counter next to your plugged-in toaster. Place a glass on the counter for milk. Keep a poured glass of juice or bowl of grapes in the fridge.
- **Oatmeal:** Place ½ cup of oats in a microwave-safe bowl and top it with a sprinkle of raisins and cinnamon. Cover the bowl with plastic wrap and leave it on the counter. Premeasure 1 cup of skim milk and leave it in the fridge. In the morning, combine oats with milk and heat on HIGH in 1-minute increments, stirring after each, until desired consistency is reached.

when to eat what

I've heard you should have an afternoon snack so you don't eat too much at dinner and the rest of the night, but I don't like fruits and veggies. What—and when—should I eat?

Having a small afternoon snack is definitely a good idea, especially when you're trying to lose weight. Without adding too many calories or spoiling your dinner, it puts a little something in your stomach between lunch and dinner to keep your hunger down so you don't overeat at the dinner table. Excluding fruits and veggies certainly puts a dent in your options, but there are still some snack ideas out there, including:

- Air-popped popcorn with a sprinkle of your favorite spice or seasoning
- A slice of multigrain bread with about a teaspoon of peanut butter or cream cheese
- 4–6 ounces yogurt
- 1 ounce baked tortilla chips
- 1 ounce pistachios or almonds
- 1 ounce reduced-fat cheese with 4 whole grain crackers
- ½ cup of whole grain cereal, dry or with ¼ cup skim milk

As far as your dislike of fruit and vegetables is concerned, I've heard this a lot when counseling people about healthy eating and weight loss. In response, I usually list about two dozen fruits and vegetables and ask my clients if they like them. They usually respond at least a few times with "Oh, I like that," and several times with "I've never had that." I firmly believe that it's impossible to dislike a food you have never tried. I challenge people in your situation to get a little creative with their fruit and vegetable habits.

First, make a conscious decision to try fruits and vegetables that are new to you. Most local grocery stores have produce sections that are simply overflowing with exotic and not-so-exotic specimens from around the globe. And when I say *try*, I mean to *really give it a good try*. Perhaps find a couple of different recipes or talk to people who like the food and try it prepared or served a few different ways before crossing it off your list. Before you limit the experiences of your taste buds, you want to make sure you've tried a food in the best possible way. Also, especially when it comes to vegetables, cooking something can result in a completely different taste experience. Until you've tried a food in a variety of different ways, you'll never know which you like best. And while there are some vegetables that you'd only want to eat cooked, such as plantain, sweet potatoes, and rhubarb, different seasoning can make a huge difference.

In addition to trying new fruits and vegetables, why not give the ones you believe you don't like another try? Don't like apples? How about baked apples with a sprinkle of brown sugar and cinnamon or a blueberry applesauce cup? Not a fan of dried apricots? Once summer hits, try a fresh one. With the multitude of flavors and textures (cooked versus raw, dried versus fresh, canned versus fresh) and the myriad spices, herbs, and other flavor enhancers available, it's hard to believe a broad statement about disliking these two food groups is based on real experience in trying them. It's not like disliking milk. With milk, what you see is what you get, with the exception of adding some flavored syrup once in a while. With produce, the taste possibilities are truly endless.

Another way to add new fruits and vegetables to your diet is to visit your local farmers' markets or join a Community Supported Agriculture Farm (CSA). Farmers' markets have been around a while, but their popularity is increasing. The number of Community Supported Agriculture Farms (CSAs) are also on the rise. Both of these venues offer tremendous opportunities to incorporate new (and more) fresh fruits and vegetables into your diet, help the environment, and try different varieties that are only available in your local area. Plus, these are beneficial to the economy and local farmers as well. To find a farmers' market in your area, go to *www.localharvest.org*.

Community Supported Agriculture Farms are a newer concept to the mainstream public. Basically, you buy a share of the farm's harvest and in return you get a portion of the harvest all season long. This is a fantastic way to try new fruits and vegetables because you've already paid for the food and you're getting a bit of everything they harvest each week—not just one or two things you request. Often the farm will give you some recipes for ways to try some of the less popular foods. There's truly no better way to eat fresh and local food. You can also find CSAs in your area through *www.localharvest.org*.

Now, just to give you an additional nudge to give veggies another try, keep in mind that they are a great addition to any diet due to their assortment of vitamins, minerals, and other nutrients—and they're especially good if you're trying to lose weight. In fact, a recent study released in the *American Journal of Clinical Nutrition* found that simply serving larger portions of vegetables at a meal resulted in more vegetables being eaten. But on top of that, when that larger serving of veggies replaced a bit of the meat or grain portion of the meal, participants ate fewer calories at the meal. And then when the added veggies had less fat added to them, the calorie intake dropped even more. Even though the amount of calories was lower, up to 17 percent lower, the amount of food eaten was the same. So if we add veggies to our meals while we cut back a bit on the meat and grain servings, we can get the same amount of food for fewer calories. This can help prevent those feelings of deprivation that often appear when you diet. So go green! And give those veggies another chance!

Occasionally, I go out to eat for a special meal and want to be able to splurge. Usually, I save up all my calories for the day, so I can eat whatever I want, but then I find that I overindulge once I'm there. What low-cal options can I eat through the day so I can enjoy my special meal without guilt, but without overindulging either?

Saving your calories up for a whopper of a meal sounds like a good idea. But it almost always backfires. A review of more than a dozen studies revealed that people who skip meals have a higher body mass index (BMI) than those who don't skip meals. For example, when you skip breakfast, you think you're pulling one over on your body, but that's not the case. Your body makes up for it by storing that hunger for later. Then when later comes, you indulge in higher-fat and calorie-dense meals, leading to weight gain.

There's nothing wrong with wanting to be able to splurge a bit when you go out to enjoy a special meal, but there's a much healthier way of going about it. Instead of eating nothing all day and leaving your body begging for food, give it food throughout the day; just make your meals and snacks lighter than usual. Cut down each meal by about a third or so and evenly across the food groups. In other words, don't just cut out all grains, or all fruits, or all protein. Aside from missing valuable nutrients, you'll miss out on the benefits each food group offers as a whole, including the energy carbs provide and the comfortable, lasting fullness protein offers. For example, if lunch is often a sandwich with an apple and some chips or cookies, keep the sandwich, choose a smaller fruit (such as a plum), and skip the chips or cookies. These small cutbacks should give you a few hundred calories to spare by the time you arrive at the restaurant.

MAKE IT WORK FOR YOU

Sure, we all know restaurant meals are a lot higher in fat and calories than the meals we cook at home. But how loaded can they really be? Many contain as much as half to well over a day's worth of calories—and multiple days' worth of heart- and artery-clogging saturated fat. Many restaurants' websites list their nutritional information. Check them out to learn more about the foods you order.

when to eat *what*

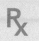

I've heard you should eat smaller meals at night and larger meals at lunch. Is this true?

There are many possible reasons why this could be useful when trying to eat healthier and lose weight. It seems to make sense to eat the largest amount of calories while you're still up and around to burn them off. Plus, by doing so, you then eat fewer calories late in the day when you're more sedentary and heading to bed. In addition, we know that people who skip meals or eat very little during the day tend to overeat later in the day and into the evening. It makes sense that a plan to eat more food earlier in the day, possibly even a bigger breakfast, would help a person to avoid overeating at night. Then all those extra, unnecessary calories are not consumed.

There's certainly no harm in eating this way, but you should make sure that this style of eating works well for your lifestyle. See how it makes you feel and if it helps you lose weight. If it does, then great—you've found what works for you. If not, chalk it up to experience and continue trying to find a healthy eating style that works best for you. The two-week menu in the back of this book is designed so that the three main meals of the day are roughly the same size. However, when you break it down, breakfast is the smallest by a bit and dinner is the largest by a bit. Feel free to flip-flop the lunch and dinner choices to see how eating your largest meal midday works for you.

When I go out for a drink with my friends, what are the best drinks to keep my weight in check and what drinks should I steer clear of?

There are so many things to consider when it comes to figure-friendly drinks: size, amount of alcohol, and mixers added to the drink. Let's start by breaking it down into the three main categories: beer, wine, and liquor.

Beer

The type of beer—regular, light, dark, and so forth—can have an impact, as can your decision to order a beer in a bottle or a draught. Bottles and cans are typically 12 ounces, whereas a beer served from a tap is usually served in a pint glass so you end up with 16 ounces. Here's the basic beer rundown:

Beer Breakdown		
Type	Calories (12 oz.)	Calories (16 oz.)
Regular	150	200
Light	110	150
Dark	175	233
Guinness	160	210

Wine

Wine is probably the least complicated choice. The biggest variable here is the size of the glass, or more specifically, the amount of wine they can put in the glass. Wine has about 85 calories a serving, but a serving of wine is about

when to eat what

3.5 ounces, just under ½ cup. When you order wine in a restaurant or bar, you're probably getting closer to a full cup of wine, which ends up being 190 calories. Instead, try ordering a wine spritzer: ask the bartender to mix half wine and half sparkling water. You'll end up with the same size drink with only half the calories.

Liquor

Liquor itself is actually pretty low in calories, only about 65 calories per ounce, but most mixed drinks contain more than 1 ounce as well as other ingredients (soda, cream, sugar syrups, juices, etc.) that can send the calories soaring. Keeping in mind that all bartenders have their own recipes and styles and that some may be a bit more heavy handed when creating their concoctions—as well as the fact that different bars serve different-sized drinks—here are some rough estimates of calories found in an average size of a few popular drinks:

Mixed Drinks	
Drink	Calories
Piña Colada	425
White Russian	420
Appletini	270
Margarita	220

Clearly, your choice of drink can make a huge difference in your nightly calorie intake. If this is a social activity you enjoy on a regular basis, a higher-calorie choice could really start to add up.

But here's some good news. Changing your behavior when you go out for a drink can actually help decrease the amount of drinks you consume. First, just set your drink down between sips. When you hold a drink in your hand, it's much easier to keep sipping and sipping until suddenly the drink's gone. Second, alternate calorie-and-alcohol-filled drinks with water or a juice spritzer (half juice, half sparkling water). Just like that, you will cut your drink consumption in half.

My day starts at 5:00. When and what should I eat for breakfast so that I can keep in line with my family's usual lunch and dinnertimes?

With such an early day you luck out—you get two breakfasts! But I wouldn't make them both the lumberjack specials unless you want to look like a lumberjack. Having both a 6:00 A.M. and a 9:00 A.M. mini breakfast should let you jump right into your family's mealtimes for the remainder of the day. For the average person, a 400-calorie breakfast works well. Depending on your appetite, you can either split this evenly or, if you're not very hungry first thing, try 100 calories early on and 300 later (or vice versa, if you're ravenous first thing). The more food groups you can include, the more well-rounded and nutrient-packed your breakfasts will be. I'd aim for at least fruit, whole grains, protein, and low-fat dairy. And if you can get some veggies in an egg dish, way to go! A few ideas to get you started include:

First meal: Mushroom, onion, and pepper omelet (made with 2 eggs); ⅓ cup strawberries
Second meal: 1 slice whole grain toast with ½ tablespoon peanut butter; 1 cup skim milk

First meal: 2 (4") pancakes topped with ⅓ cup blueberries; 1 cup skim milk
Second meal: 1 medium banana; ¾ cup low-fat yogurt

First meal: 1 multigrain English muffin topped with an all-fruit spread; ½ cup 100% fruit juice
Second meal: 2 hardboiled eggs; 1 cup diced melon

But don't limit yourself to these ideas; look at the labels of some of your own favorite breakfast foods and figure out how you can turn them into a two-breakfast special.

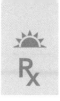

My stomach tends to get upset. What can I eat for breakfast to keep it calm throughout my day?

Yogurt can be a great part of a healthy breakfast—especially for those with digestive issues. Why? The presence of live active cultures. Look on the label to make sure yours contain them. These cultures, called probiotics, work to improve the health and function of the digestive system. We actually have bacteria in our intestinal tract, and probiotics help to keep them in the proper balance. Probiotics can be helpful when dealing with a bout of diarrhea, and they can help combat some of the common intestinal side effects of antibiotics, such as gas, bloating, and diarrhea. Antibiotics kill all bacteria, even the good guys, and that's what leads to those unpleasant side effects. Probiotics help to replace what gets destroyed and, in doing so, can alleviate those symptoms.

As healthy as yogurt is for us, you need to be careful about what type you choose. It can make a big difference on the amount of calories and added sugar you get. When yogurt first hit the market years ago, you had one choice: plain. Fast forward several dozen years, and you can get anything from cinnamon bun and key lime pie yogurts to yogurt with mini candy bits or granola to mix in. Some 6-ounce containers have more than 7 teaspoons or 28 grams of sugar and close to 200 calories, which seems like more of a dessert than a healthy snack or breakfast option. In fact, these really aren't bad *dessert choices*, because they give you a dose of protein and calcium. However, if you enjoy yogurt as part of a healthy breakfast or a snack, your best bet is to buy fat-free plain or vanilla yogurt and mix in real fruit. This way you save a ton of calories and sugar but get the added bonus of a serving of fruit.

I've read that fiber is great to eat when you're trying to lose weight, but I have celiac disease and can't eat gluten. How can I get enough fiber and lose weight when I can't eat whole wheat?

Whole wheat is certainly a major contributor of fiber, but you don't have to eat whole wheat to meet your daily fiber needs. Fruits and vegetables are good sources of fiber, and they are also a valued inclusion to any weight-loss diet due to their low calorie and fat content and their high water content. Oats are also a great source of fiber, but there has been some controversy about whether oats should be included in a gluten-free diet. The latest consensus is that a small amount of pure, uncontaminated oats is safe for most people with celiac disease. If you don't currently eat oats, speak to your doctor or dietitian before adding them to your diet.

The food that can provide you with the biggest fiber boost is beans, which contain about 7 grams of fiber per ½ cup; on top of that they're a great source of lean protein. Beans are nutritious, inexpensive, and versatile, so feel free to add them to chilis, soups, and stews. They can be used in salads, dips, and spreads, as well as wraps. Believe it or not, you can even mash them and add them to brownies and cookies. You can also use bean flour in place of other flours when you bake. This is definitely one of those glass-half-full situations. While you may not be able to eat whole wheat foods, there are still plenty of high-fiber foods you can include in your diet.

MAKE IT WORK FOR YOU

With the rise of gluten-free products on the market, as well as books about gluten-free diets popping up on bookstore shelves, it seems that gluten free is the way to go. However, by choosing to follow such a diet without the advice or follow-up of a medical professional, you could be putting yourself at risk of nutritional deficiencies. If you believe you have celiac disease or a gluten intolerance, do not self-diagnose. Make an appointment with your healthcare professional to discuss your concerns.

when to eat *what*

I have to admit it: I reach for the salt shaker before I even taste my food! I just want to taste some flavor, especially if I'm not eating as much as before. Is it better for my diet to substitute sea salt for regular table salt?

Americans are so used to eating salt that many believe that in order for food to taste good, it has to taste salty. It's really sad that so many people miss out on the wonderful flavors nature gives us because they are so accustomed to salt that their ability to taste and savor the true flavors of foods has greatly diminished. In the minds and mouths of many Americans, flavor/taste equals salt.

Excess salt can increase your risk of developing hypertension or high blood pressure, which in turn can increase your risk of having a stroke or heart attack. Additionally, if you're trying to lose weight, eating too much sodium is going to put a kink in your plans.

Sodium and fluids have a very close relationship in the human body; they must be kept in the proper balance for your various organs and systems to work correctly. A simple explanation is that the sodium levels in your body need to be kept at around a certain percentage or concentration in the water in your body. When you eat too much salt, that concentration goes up. To counteract this, your body begins to hold on to extra water in an attempt to bring the sodium concentration down to the proper levels. Water isn't weightless. In fact, one gallon of water weighs just over 8 pounds. Chances are you're not carrying around an extra gallon of water, but

MAKE IT WORK FOR YOU

You're trying to cut back on sodium, so those little jars of substitutes next to the canisters of salt are perfect, right? Not so fast. There are two types of salt substitutes. The first are the ones labeled light or lite. These actually do still contain some sodium. The second type of salt substitute replaces sodium with the mineral potassium. For many people, these are fine salt replacements; however, you should check with your doctor before using them. Potassium could possibly be dangerous if you have any kidney problems.

if you're regularly eating too much salt, there's a good chance you're lugging around at least a few extra pounds.

If you're ready to shake the salt habit, there are several ways to go about it. The first—and easiest—is to decrease the amount of sodium you actually add to food. There are a few ways to accomplish this. One involves taping over a few of the holes on your salt shaker so less salt comes out. If you tend to shake just out of habit, this little trick can help. Another trick is to leave the salt out of your food when you're cooking, but still allow yourself to shake at the table. Because you're putting the salt right on top of your meal, you'll taste it much more strongly than any salt that would have been added during cooking, plus you'll save whatever you didn't add in.

If you want to stop using salt entirely, there is a huge assortment of various salt-free seasonings in the spice aisle. McCormick has a line, and Mrs. Dash Salt-Free Seasoning Blends has fifteen different varieties. Flavors include the old standbys of garlic and herb, lemon and pepper, and Italian medley, as well as more exotic and unique flavor mixtures such as fiesta lime and southwest chipotle. These seasonings provide intense flavor without any sodium whatsoever. Also, adding dried herbs as you cook can boost the flavor without adding salt. Try basil, oregano, rosemary, thyme, and more.

You can also look beyond the jar to flavor your foods. Sautéed garlic, shallots, and onions can really add a flavor punch, as can fresh ginger and herbs like parsley, basil, and chives. And, keep some fresh lemons on hand. A squeeze of fresh lemon juice brightens up a dish and can make the taste pop. When you look at all these options, I'd say you're just limiting yourself by using only salt.

MAKE IT WORK FOR YOU

It looks like garlic may do much more than just add delicious flavor to your meals. Its potential health benefits have been researched for years with positive results. A review of current data on garlic and heart health shows that the little bulb may be beneficial in protecting against heart disease. Garlic has also been shown to improve blood cholesterol levels, blood protein levels, and more.

when to eat what

You mention using sea salt. Because the process of obtaining sea salt is all natural, it's often perceived as a healthier alternative than ordinary table salt. In reality, it's still salt, and by weight it contains the same amount of sodium as table salt. However, like kosher salt, sea salt's granules are much larger, which means there is less sodium per teaspoon. In fact, you can save about 400 milligrams of sodium using a teaspoon of kosher or sea salt instead of table salt. Since sea salt is more expensive than kosher salt but their sodium content is about the same, I'd recommend kosher salt as a substitute for table salt. If you switch from table salt to kosher salt and follow any of the other tricks I've mentioned, you will be well on your way to lowering your sodium intake.

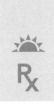

I overdid it at the all-you-can-eat buffet last night. I feel bloated and I'm sure I put on a few pounds. What can I eat to feel better?

MAKE IT WORK FOR YOU

Brightly colored berries such as strawberries, raspberries, and blueberries are good sources of a phytochemical called *anthocyanidins*. While it's too early to say that these foods will prevent certain disease, the research so far is promising. Anthocyanidins have been shown in multiple studies to have anti-cancer and anti-inflammatory proper-ties and to improve the health of blood vessels, which could lower your risk of cardiovas-cular disease.

First, the good news: the chances that you gained a few pounds are pretty slim, though it may feel like that this morning. To gain just 1 pound, you would have needed to eat 3,500 calories beyond your daily needs. However, there's a good likelihood that you did eat a large amount of fatty and salty foods, so let's counteract that first. High amounts of these foods can cause bloating and constipation, so Step One is to drink enough fluids and eat enough fiber throughout the rest of the day. Strive for around 8 to 10 glasses of water. In addition, be sure to include a good dose of fiber at every meal—fresh fruits and vegetables, whole grains, and beans all make terrific choices.

Step Two is to eat healthfully throughout the day. You may feel like you should skip a few meals to make up for the excess calories from last night, but that's one of the worst things you can do. Skipping meals will only make you overly hungry later in the day, which will probably lead you to overeat. Then you may wake up feeling the same way tomorrow!

Instead, eat well-balanced, moderately sized meals and snacks throughout the day. For example, try a meal plan like this for the day:

Breakfast: 2 slices whole grain toast topped with an all-fruit spread; 8 ounces skim milk; 1 cup strawberries; coffee or tea, if you like

Snack #1: Low-fat yogurt with ½ cup raspberries

Lunch: 2 cups spinach salad with assorted veggies; 4 to 6 whole grain crackers; 8 ounces skim milk; 1 banana

Snack #2: 1 medium apple with 1 tablespoons of peanut butter and a few raisins

Dinner: 4 ounces boneless, skinless chicken breast, grilled; 1 baked sweet potato; 1 cup steamed broccoli

Finally, you can make up for a bit of the extra indulging with an extra bit of exercising: go for a brisk thirty-minute walk, do yard work or shoveling (depending on the weather), or try some old-fashioned calisthenics (jumping jacks, running in place, jumping rope, etc.).

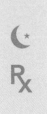

I am typically awake until at least midnight. Around 10:00, I start to feel as though I am starving. Is there anything I can eat at this time of night that does not immediately turn into fat?

It makes perfect sense for you to be hungry; it's probably been three or four hours since dinner, and that's about the time it takes for our bodies to use up a meal. It would seem, however, that you're familiar with that old rumor that any food eaten after 6:00 P.M. (or 7:00 or 8:00, depending on your version of the rumor) turns to fat as soon as we eat it. Well, the good news is that while there is a nugget of truth here, as is often the case with rumors, depending on the situation, it doesn't always work this way.

Basically, our bodies need a certain amount of calories every day to make all of our parts work properly. Everyone's needs are different based on a variety of factors, including age, height, weight, gender, activity level, and more. For simplicity's sake, let's just say we're talking about a person who needs 2,000 calories a day. Now if that person eats all of the necessary 2,000 calories by 7:00 P.M., then any additional calories eaten after 7:00 will most likely be stored as fat, since they are not needed for the day. However, if that same person eats only 1,700 calories by 10:00 P.M., then she or he could potentially eat another 300 calories without them being turned to fat.

That being said, if you're often up at this time of night, I'd start by planning a healthy 10:00 P.M. snack into your eating plan. This will allow you to satisfy that hunger without going overboard on your calorie intake every night. At this time of night,

MAKE IT WORK FOR YOU

Did you know inadequate sleep can also cause you to eat more? A small study recently found that when participants cut their evening sleep from 8.5 hours to 5.5 hours, they ate about 200 more calories a day. Those calories were primarily consumed between 7:00 P.M. and 7:00 A.M. and were from snacks, not meals. These extra calories could easily add up to a whopping 20 pounds of extra weight per year that you could potentially keep off just by going to bed a couple of hours earlier.

when to eat *what*

the best type of snack is something mild, light, and somewhat long lasting. In other words, you don't want to eat something spicy or heavy that could keep you from sleeping well. And, foods that are digested quickly like fruit by itself, candy, pastries, and so forth may satisfy you in the moment, but then your body will come down from the sugar rush—most likely when you're asleep—and you will probably wake up feeling overly hungry and sluggish. If that happens, you'll probably grab whatever food you can find quickly, which means you may end up starting your day with poor food choices.

Make sure to leave yourself enough daily calories for a late-night snack, and then try some of these options:

- 1 cup whole grain cereal with skim or 1% milk
- Whole grain crackers with 1 ounce cheese
- Nonfat plain or vanilla yogurt with 1 piece of fruit

Some snacks to stay away from include:

- Candy
- Buffalo wings
- Mexican food
- Pastries
- Sugary cereal

R_X I've had high cholesterol for years and have cut down on a lot of foods to help keep it under control, but it's hard for me to cut down on chocolate. I've recently heard that chocolate is good for you. Is it true? If so, what and how much can I eat to keep my cholesterol and weight down?

A lot of research has been done on chocolate in recent years. And the findings are good news indeed. Cocoa contains polyphenols. These are the substances similar to those found in red wine, tea, and fruits and vegetables that make them what many call superfoods, or foods that provide health benefits beyond the basic energy, vitamins, and minerals. The polyphenols in cocoa are called flavanols. They're believed to be the reason behind the multiple health benefits cocoa or chocolate seems to provide. Many of these health benefits are related to heart health and include a reduction in blood clotting, which can lower one's risk of having a heart attack or a stroke. Other benefits are improvements in blood pressure as well as blood cholesterol levels.

However, chocolate does contain calories and fat, even if it has been shown to offer cardiovascular benefits. The trick is finding out how much chocolate you can eat to obtain the benefits—along with, of course, the pure pleasure of eating chocolate—without packing on the pounds. Researchers at Syracuse University found that when participants ate about 1½ ounces of chocolate a day, along with a low-fat, calorie-controlled diet, they didn't gain weight. So as long as we factor the fat and calories into our diet, we can enjoy chocolate without weight gain—and potentially with weight loss.

It's important to note that most of the research regarding chocolate has focused on dark chocolate or cocoa. This is important information because other chocolates have added sugars, milk, and other ingredients that can alter the amount of the calories and healthful fat, and therefore its impact on weight. In addition, those extra ingredients take the place of some of the health-helping polyphenols.

All of this means that eating the same amount of milk chocolate as dark chocolate or cocoa will give you fewer benefits but more calories. How many additional calories? See the following chart:

Types of Chocolate (per 1 oz.)			
Chocolate	Calories	Sugar (in grams)	Fat (in grams)
Cocoa powder (not hot chocolate mix)	85	0	3
Dark chocolate	135	12	10
Semisweet chocolate	142	14	9
Milk chocolate	150	15	8

On the weekends I have more time to cook. What can I eat for a more nutritious breakfast?

Your first step should be to consider all the food groups and how you can get as many as possible into a meal. Breakfast foods in general tend to include at least three of the five major food groups—grain, fruit, dairy—but lean protein and veggies can be fit in fairly easily. The following are just a few foods from each group that you can easily incorporate in a healthy breakfast:

Food Group	Foods
Grain	whole grain bread/toast, whole grain English muffins, whole grain cereals, oatmeal, bagels, waffles, pancakes, French toast
Fruit	fresh fruit such as berries, bananas, melon, and more; unsweetened frozen fruit to add to smoothies; 100% fruit juice
Dairy	skim or 1% milk, nonfat yogurt, reduced-fat cheese for egg dishes
Lean Protein	eggs, peanut butter, tofu, ham
Vegetables	onions, peppers, tomato, spinach, broccoli for egg dishes
Healthy Fat	nuts, avocado

Here are a few meal ideas to get you started:

- **Florentine eggs:** Scramble 1 or 2 eggs in a small, nonstick skillet. When they're almost set, add 2 tablespoons reduced-fat shredded cheese and ¼ to ½ cup frozen spinach, thawed and squeezed dry. Fold all together just long enough to melt cheese and heat spinach. Serve with a piece of whole grain toast and an orange or ½ cup orange juice.
- **Pumpkin pancakes:** Follow the directions for pancakes on your favorite regular or whole grain baking mix or pancake mix box. For every 2 cups mix, add ⅔ cup canned puréed pumpkin (not pumpkin pie mix), ½ teaspoon vanilla extract, 1 teaspoon cinnamon, ½ teaspoon ginger, and ½ teaspoon nutmeg. Prepare according to recipe. Serve with 1 cup of skim milk and 1 banana, sliced.

when to eat what

- **Egg sandwich:** Toast a whole grain English muffin. Scramble or fry 1 egg in a nonstick pan. Place egg on ½ the muffin. Top with 1 slice of reduced-fat cheese, 1 slice of tomato, 1 slice of avocado, and the top half of the muffin. You could also add a slice of ham or Canadian bacon if you like. Serve with 1 cup grapes.
- **French toast:** Use 3 slices whole grain bread and dunk in a mixture of 1 large egg, 3 tablespoons skim milk, a dash of vanilla, and a sprinkle of cinnamon. Cook as usual. Serve with a blueberry sauce made by simmering frozen blueberries, a bit of water, lemon juice, and sugar in a small saucepan over medium-low heat, stirring and mashing as necessary, until it thickens slightly.

Since your weekday mornings are a bit more rushed, consider making these ideas serve double duty. Make extras on the weekend and use them during the week. For pancakes, French toast, or waffles, let them cool completely in a single layer. Then place them in an airtight container or zipper bag, with a sheet of waxed paper between each. Store them in the fridge for a couple of days or in the freezer for a couple of months. For weekday breakfasts, take out one serving and heat it in a skillet over medium heat or in your toaster.

For make-ahead breakfast sandwiches, leave off the tomato and avocado. Wrap sandwiches individually in waxed paper or aluminum foil. Refrigerate for no more than 1 week without ham or 3 to 4 days with ham. When ready to heat, simply unwrap and zap in the microwave for 20 to 30 seconds, or until the cheese starts to melt.

MAKE IT WORK FOR YOU

Pumpkin is an excellent source of the carotenoid beta carotene, which has been linked to a possible reduction in risk of various cancers, including breast and cervical. It's important to obtain valuable nutrients like carotenoids from real foods versus supplements. Fortunately canned pumpkin purée (not pie filling) makes adding pumpkin, and thus beta carotene, to your diet fairly easy. Pumpkin purée can be added to pancake, quick bread, and muffin batters; oatmeal; soups; and more.

I'm concerned about the environment. How can I eat in a "green" fashion and still lose weight?

Your two aims actually work together quite well. Many of the changes you can make in your food habits to eat green are also great dieting and weight-loss tips. For example, rethinking your drink can make a huge impact on the environment, especially if your fridge is filled with bottled waters, sodas, fruit drinks, sports drinks, and other caloric or noncaloric drinks. America's landfills are filled with these bottles. Tap water is the drink with the least impact on both your waistline and the environment. Instead of buying and discarding bottle after bottle of assorted drinks, switch to tap water and buy a couple of the reusable bottles to carry around with you. If you're not crazy about the taste of your water, there are plenty of inexpensive filters available.

In addition, try the following options:

- Cut down on the amount of red meat that you eat. Many red meats are high in fat and calories, and cutting back a bit will certainly help promote weight loss. It's also very costly, environmentally speaking, to get red meat from the farm to your table. Twice a week, try having a meat-free meal. Tofu, beans, and pasta all make great bases for delicious and healthy meals.
- "Brown bag" your lunch—except use nylon or neoprene bags that you can reuse. Skip the plastic wrap and foil and invest in a few reusable containers in which you can pack your leftovers, sandwiches, cut up veggies, and fruit. A homemade lunch is far more likely to be lower in fat, calories, and sodium (and higher in fiber, vitamins, and minerals) than one you have to buy when you're at work.
- Say no to supersizing. Sure, the popcorn vat at the movies is only 50 cents more than the kiddie size, but it's far more costly in the long run. The same principle applies when grocery shopping. The 5-pound crate of strawberries is only economical and environmentally friendly if you'll actually use them all before they spoil. Try buying just what you need to avoid overeating and wasting food.

- Snack smarter. It's easy to buy the single-serving boxes of cookies, crackers, even cut-up carrot sticks. But in a week's time you'll wind up eating more processed foods than you really should if you're trying to lose weight. Plus your garbage will be filled with dozens of single-serving pouches, bags, and boxes. Instead, focus more on whole foods and less on processed foods, and buy multiserving packages and portion out your own.
- Eat locally and seasonally. Try hitting the farmers' market once every week or so. The more fresh produce you have in the house, the more fresh produce you're likely to eat. Buying more local and in-season foods uses far less fuel and energy to store and transport than the same food from across the country or around the world.

What can I eat besides salad every day for lunch? Our cafeteria offers burgers, pizza, and sandwiches along with a salad bar, but salad day after day can get boring.

It's great that your cafeteria has a salad bar, but eating the same thing day after day can understandably lead to boredom. Mixing up what you eat is a great step in helping you stick to your diet and achieve your weight-loss goals. In this case, I would suggest customizing your salad each day by bringing some add-ins from home. Remember, a well-balanced salad does more for you than just taste good and keep calories in check. Salad greens are a great source of the antioxidants lutein and zeaxanthin, and multiple studies have confirmed that these two antioxidants help reduce your risk of developing age-related macular degeneration (ARMD), the leading cause of blindness in older Americans. The highest dietary sources of these nutrients are green vegetables (including broccoli, kale, spinach, Brussels sprouts, and collard greens), along with corn, tangerines, and nectarines—items commonly found in, you guessed it, salads.

So pair your cafeteria's salad bar items with foods you bring from home in a small cooler and you can have a deliciously different yet still healthy salad each day. Try the following suggestions to create a unique salad sensation:

Type of Salad	Toppings
Greek	black olives, reduced-fat feta cheese, spinach, Greek dressing; serve with a small whole grain pita
Californian	diced avocado, bean sprouts, walnuts, red wine vinaigrette
Latin	black beans, corn, pineapple tidbits, cilantro, reduced-fat Cheddar-jack cheese, hot peppers, lime-based dressing
Asian	mushrooms, scallions, tofu, sesame seeds, chow mein noodles, soy-based dressing
Italian	cooked whole grain rotini pasta, spinach, reduced-fat mozzarella cheese, pepperoni or salami (just a tiny bit for flavor), basil, olive oil and red wine vinegar dressing

when to eat *what*

Use these options as a springboard for your own creativity. Perhaps bring in some crusty whole grain bread or whole grain crackers, yogurt, and a different type of fruit each day to spice things up. Whatever you decide to do, be sure to play off of your favorite types of foods and flavor combinations to come up with more ways to dress a simple salad.

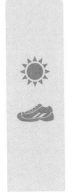

I don't have time to worry about making a lunch, so I usually just buy a week's worth of frozen meals that I bring in to work on Monday. Am I spoiling all my healthy eating by having these for lunch five days a week? How can I make sure the ones I pick won't lead to weight gain? Are there things I can do to make them a bit healthier?

Frozen meals won't necessarily spoil your healthy eating. Indeed, they can certainly fit into a healthy diet, and can even help with weight loss. The good news first: a University of Illinois study followed participants who either prepared their own meals using the Food Pyramid guidelines or chose from an assortment of twenty-four different prepackaged frozen meals for eight weeks. Both groups aimed to get about 1,700 calories a day. At the end of the study, those eating the frozen meals lost an average of 5 pounds more than those who prepared their own meals. Researchers suspect the biggest reason for this difference is that the frozen meals were automatically portion controlled. They left little to no room for overeating a little here or there. No extra spoonful of potatoes or slices of meat.

The bad news: processed foods, including frozen meals, are notoriously high in sodium. In fact, some meals can contain a half a day's worth or more. In addition, many frozen meals are jam-packed with fat and calories. And, to make matters worse, they are often lacking in whole grains, fruits, and vegetables. Often, the one or two slivers of carrot you may see on the front label is what they consider the veggie part of the meal. However, all hope is not lost. There are several brands on the market that cater to a healthier/lower calorie lifestyle, such as Healthy Choice and Weight Watchers Smart Ones.

when to eat *what*

If you want to include frozen meals as part of your regular diet due to convenience or the portion-control assistance, here are a few pointers to keep in mind:

- **Aim for around 300 to 400 calories.** If you eat less than this, you're likely not getting enough calories to get you through to snack time let alone your next meal. You could also end up slowing your metabolism down by consistently eating too little. Much more and you risk getting too much fat and calories for one meal.
- **Try to find meals with less than 700 milligrams of sodium.** If it's difficult in your market, try to get as close to that as possible.
- **Balance out your meals.** Add a glass of skim milk, a piece of fruit, and perhaps a small salad to make up for the low veggie content.

My coworkers and I go to happy hour a few times a week. But between the greasy munchies and the drinks, I end up feeling bloated and uncomfortable afterward. Plus, my weight is creeping up! What can I eat to still be a part of the group but keep my health in check?

High-calorie drinks, alcohol-induced reduced inhibitions, and fatty and salty snacks are not a recipe for a night of fitness and nutrition. However, there's no argument that socializing with friends and relaxing are key components to a healthy lifestyle. The trick is finding how you can mesh some healthy habits in with the happy hour scene to make it a win-win for your waistline and your social life. Two important rules: 1) Don't go out with an empty stomach. 2) Consume fewer high-calorie drinks. Let's get Rule 2 out of the way. I know it's not rocket science, but cutting back on high-calorie drinks—or cutting out alcoholic beverages altogether—really can make a difference. To take a look at the amount of calories found in popular drinks, take another look at the chart under entry "When I go out for a drink with my friends, what are the best drinks to keep my weight in check and what drinks should I steer clear of?"

As far as Rule 1 is concerned, when you're hungry, your resistance to spicy wings, gooey mozzarella sticks, and crunchy nachos is at an all-time low. Add to that the fact that researchers have shown that alcohol stimulates the appetite. This leads people who are drinking to eat more. In addition, high-fat, salty foods are the foods most chosen in these situations. What's in these happy hour snacks, you ask? Here's a rough breakdown of a few favorites:

Snack	Calories	Fat in grams	Sodium in milligrams
¼ order of chicken nachos	505	28	745
½ order of serving mini chicken quesadillas	325	14	545
3 fried mozzarella sticks	307	18	761
¼ order of artichoke spinach dip	302	18	520
5 fried buffalo wings	250	12	877

when to eat what

Keep in mind these numbers are just the appetizer and do not include the sour cream, blue cheese, or other dips you may add to your food.

So before you head out, make sure you eat at least a little something. Pack a pre–happy hour snack to bring to work with you and have it just before you clock out. A few good snacks for this situation would be:

- 1 ounce of your favorite nuts
- 1 small peanut butter sandwich on whole grain bread
- 1 ounce of reduced-fat cheese with 4 to 6 whole grain crackers
- A couple of spoonfuls of hummus with baby carrots

Also, have a glass of skim milk, water, or other low-calorie or calorie-free drink before you head out to the bar. If you walk in thirsty, gulping down a beer or mixed drink to quench that thirst already has you starting off on the wrong foot.

MAKE IT WORK FOR YOU

Obviously, having a designated driver is a potentially lifesaving plan when going out drinking. But volunteering for that important job once or twice a week may also save you hundreds of calories: the ones in the alcoholic drink and the ones you might have been tempted to consume when the alcohol made your appetite swell.

I find my mind gets cloudy and my energy usually bottoms out by 1:30 or 2:00 P.M. What are some healthy, energy-boosting snacks I can eat to get me through the rest of the work day?

In this situation, a lot of people rush to the vending machine to grab a candy bar, go to the local coffee shop for a little buzz, or both. Unfortunately, all of those solutions, if you can call them that, are probably the worst things you can do. The sugar in the candy, like the caffeine in the coffee, only give you an immediate, short-lasting burst of energy. But what goes up must come down, and from these kinds of sudden energy shots, the resulting low is often lower than where you started in the first place.

Take a two-pronged approach to this problem. First, plan an early afternoon to mid-afternoon snack to counteract the afternoon slump. I say *plan* because in many instances this involves foods you must bring from home. Otherwise, you may hit the vending machine a bit too often. And when it comes to planning a snack in this situation, you have to tackle the issue from both sides. Yes, you need that quick rush of energy to help you now, but you also don't want to find yourself in the same situation in a few hours, so be sure you include some slower-release foods too.

Good snacks for this time of day include:

- Pistachios and dried cranberries
- Cashews and raisins
- Reduced-fat cheese and whole grain crackers
- Low-fat yogurt and fruit

The second prong follows the old saying that prevention is the best medicine. Eating lunch is crucial to help prevent the afternoon lull. But the real key is what that lunch is made up of. A 150-calorie frozen meal, a small salad, or a yogurt with some fruit can all be great components of a satisfying lunch, but if you're only eating *one* of them as your whole meal, it's time for a change.

You first want to make sure you're taking in enough calories for lunch. For the average person on a 1,600- to 2,000-calorie diet, that means around 400 to 500 calories. You also want to make sure those calories come from foods that will satisfy you and keep you satisfied for three to four hours. For that, you need fiber and protein. Both of these nutrients take longer to digest than carbohydrates and therefore keep you feeling fuller longer. To help create a healthy, long-lasting lunch, try choosing at least one food from each of the columns in this table:

Whole Grains	Lean Protein	Fruit/Veggies	Low-Fat Dairy
whole wheat pasta	egg	greens	skim milk
whole grain crackers	lean meat	baby carrots	low-fat yogurt
whole grain breads	peanut butter	apple slices	reduced-fat cheese
whole grain cereals	tofu	berries	
brown rice	nuts	applesauce cup	
	water-packed tuna	bell pepper strips	

I need my morning cup of java to get my day started, but I like it sweet. What's the best way to sweeten my coffee—sugar, honey, Sweet'N Low, stevia, agave nectar, or something else?

A lot of this depends on your personal tastes as well as what you're looking for (low- or no-calorie, all natural, etc.). Here's a chart to help explain the differences:

Sweeteners (per 2 teaspoons)			
Sweetener	Calories	Natural or Artificial?	Glycemic Index
Sugar	32	Natural	70
Stevia	0	Natural	0
Honey	40	Natural	55
Agave nectar	40	Natural	30
Sweet'N Low (Saccharin)	0	Artificial	0
Splenda (Sucralose)	0	Artificial	0
NutraSweet (Aspartame)	0	Artificial	0

A couple of the items in the chart are pretty self-explanatory. If calories are your concern, you can make your choice accordingly. If you prefer natural to artificial, again, you can easily narrow your options. The final column, however, may need a bit more explaining.

The glycemic index is a measure of how quickly a food, drink, or in this case a sweetener, raises your blood sugar. If you happen to be feeling symptoms of low blood sugar—fatigue, light-headedness, hunger—then something that raises your blood sugar quickly may be just what you need. In that case, select something with a higher glycemic index. In addition, if you're exercising for a short period of time and you need a little boost to get you through, a quick blood sugar rise could help you out. If, on the other hand, you're getting ready

when to eat what

to be active or start your day, you may be better off with something that raises your blood sugar slowly and steadily versus a quick rise and fall.

As for the natural-versus-artificial sweetener argument, when you're trying to lose weight, the no-calorie sweeteners may seem like a no-brainer, but it may not be that simple. There's conflicting research on whether artificial or no-calorie sweeteners are beneficial to or harmful to weight loss. One would assume they would be an ideal ingredient in a low-calorie weight loss diet because you can eat or drink the foods or beverages the sweeteners are found in with little to no calories. Well, maybe. There is some research to show that when we eat these artificial and no-calorie sweeteners, our body stops linking the sweet taste with calories. This can interfere with calorie-intake regulation, so you may actually eat or drink more calories when you use these sweeteners than you would eat or drink if you just used sugar, honey, or some other caloric sweetener.

I'm going on a cruise soon and I'm nervous about the food. I've heard there's food available 24 hours a day for the length of the cruise. When and what should I eat so I won't need a new wardrobe when I get home?

There is an awful lot of food available on cruises. The good news is that it's not all loaded with fat, calories, and sugar. In fact, quite a bit of it is healthy. There's usually no end to the amount of fresh fruit available, and it's often a bit more exotic than you're likely used to seeing at home. In addition, dinner usually always includes one or more seafood options. So instead of thinking, "How can I *not* overeat?" why not look at it as an opportunity to try some new healthy foods? Make a rule that every time you eat, half of your plate will be fruits and vegetables, which have a high water content. A large body of scientific evidence has shown that eating meals with a lower-energy density—which are foods of which you can eat large portions for only a small amount of calories—are related to healthier diets, lower calorie intake, and lower body weight. Low-energy density foods include those with a high water content such as fruits and vegetables. While doing this, continue, of course, to choose lean foods as much as possible—grilled chicken, baked potato, and so forth. That's not to say that you won't or can't splurge once in a while over the course of your vacation, but if you can eat healthy and well-balanced meals 80 to 90 percent of the time, it'll make the other 10 or 20 percent of the time not as significant.

You can also cut back on food intake by not eating at every eating occasion. It's not as hard as it seems. I don't mean you should skip regular meals, but on cruise ships there is always food available somewhere. Fortunately, cruise ships are huge, so it is fairly easy to position yourself away from the sixth buffet of the day when it's only 2:00 in the afternoon. On top of that, there are so many activities on board, you're bound to find plenty to keep you busy that doesn't involve food. Explore a port of call; check out a magic show, comedy show, Broadway musical; or gamble at the casino. And to make up for those occasional splurges, take advantage of the ship's track and go for a brisk morning walk, sign up for a yoga or aerobics class, or check out the ship's fitness room.

when to eat what

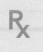

R_X **I just had a baby and have gained a bit more weight than I should. What can I eat to help me lose the extra baby weight?**

Losing baby weight requires a healthy diet. I'll get to the basics of that, but first here is some important information for breastfeeding moms. If you are breast-feeding, do not try to restrict calories in any way until your milk supply is fully in. You want to make sure your body has the calories and nutrients it needs to pro-duce enough nutritious milk for your little one. This usually takes about twelve weeks. In addition, multiple studies have shown that breastfeeding mothers have increased postpartum weight loss compared to the mothers of babies who were exclusively formula fed. In fact, a recent study in the *American Journal of Clinical Nutrition* found that at both six months and eighteen months after deliv-ery, the breastfeeding moms had lost more of their baby weight. In fact, based on these results, researchers predicted that women who gained right around 26 pounds during their pregnancy and then breastfed exclusively for six months would lose all of their pregnancy weight in that same time period. They found this to be true in all women except for the extremely overweight. Coincidently, this same time frame—six months—is what the American Academy of Pediatrics recommends as the minimum women should try to exclusively breastfeed their babies to gain the greatest health benefits for the baby. In addition, the action of breastfeeding, specifically the baby's sucking, triggers a hormone to be released in the mother that helps shrink the uterus back to normal size faster.

It's important to note that breastfeeding requires an additional 500 calories more than your usual prepregnancy intake, each day. So pay attention to this when eating. If you notice your milk supply is diminishing once you start to cut your calories, make sure you're eating enough food and drinking enough flu-ids. The good news is that you shouldn't need to force fluids; simply pay close attention to your body and be sure to answer whenever it tells you it's thirsty. A good practice is to put a big glass of your favorite uncaffeinated, nonalcoholic drink within your reach every time you prepare to nurse. This shouldn't be hard to remember, though. For many women, the act of nursing makes you thirsty, especially in the beginning.

Even if you're not breastfeeding, you need to be sure you eat enough throughout the day to keep you strong enough to take care of your new little family member. Everyone's caloric needs differ depending on their height, weight, age, and activity level, so it's impossible to give one generic diet that will work for everyone. What I like to do is recommend a range of servings from each food group along with examples of what is in each food group to help you find out what works best for you.

Food Group	Number of Daily Servings	Serving Size/ Examples	Tip
Dairy	3–4	8 oz. milk; 8 oz. yogurt; ½ cup soft cheese (cottage or ricotta); ⅓ cup shredded cheese; 1 oz. hard cheese	Choose low fat, reduced fat, nonfat, or skim
Fruit	3–4	1 medium piece; ½ banana or grapefruit; ½ cup frozen, canned, chopped, or small fruit; 2 tablespoons dried; ½ cup 100% juice	Limit juice to 1 serving per day and if choosing canned fruit, get packed in juice, not syrup
Vegetables	4–5	½ cup cooked fresh, frozen, or canned; 1 cup raw; ½ cup juice	Vegetable juices can be high in sodium, so look for low-sodium varieties
Grains, Beans, Starchy Veggies	5–8	1 slice bread; 1 cup dry cereal; ½ cup hot cooked cereal, oatmeal, pasta, or rice; 3 cups popcorn (light microwave or air popped); ½ cup corn, peas, or potatoes; ½ cup beans (such as black, kidney, red, pinto)	Choose whole grains such as brown rice and whole grain breads, cereals, and pastas for at least half of your daily servings

when to eat what

Food Group	Number of Daily Servings	Serving Size/ Examples	Tip
Lean Protein	2–3	3 oz. lean chicken, beef, pork, seafood; 3 oz. tofu; 1 egg; ¼ cup of egg replacement; 1 serving of a soy-based meat replacement (soy dogs, burgers, crumbles); 1 tablespoons peanut butter or other nut butters; 1 oz. nuts	If eating 3 servings per day, choose at least one nonanimal source of protein
Fat	3	1 teaspoon butter or margarine; 1 tablespoon reduced-fat mayonnaise or salad dressings; 2½ teaspoons canola or olive oil; ⅓ avocado; ¼ cup or 2 oz. dark chocolate	Choose the healthier fats more often, such as canola or olive oil and avocado

In addition, take advantage of your baby's naps to catch up on your own rest. Midnight feedings can take their toll, so it's important to nap while the baby naps. Believe it or not, you need to get adequate sleep to lose weight. Studies show that with inadequate sleep, the levels of the hormones insulin and cortisol in your body increase. Such elevated levels can stand in the way of losing weight.

Also, don't forget that exercise is crucial to losing weight healthfully, too. As soon as your doctor allows you to resume exercising (roughly six weeks after giving birth), start taking daily walks to begin burning some extra calories. Bring the baby along in either a stroller or a chest-style baby carrier. The added weight will create extra resistance when you walk, which increases the calories you burn. Plus, the baby will probably like the steady, rhythmic motion and may even drift off for a snooze.

I went out for drinks with friends and overdid it. What can I eat right now to sober up that won't completely ruin my diet?

Okay, so despite your good intentions, you've found yourself more inebriated than planned. Now, how to sober up? Cold shower? Hot coffee? Unfortunately, none of the methods you see in the movies work in real life. The only way to sober up is to let the alcohol get out of your bloodstream. That's not to say you can't help it along a bit, but don't expect anything you do to suddenly turn your tumbling, slurring, and tripping into walking a straight line and saying the alphabet backwards.

Next time, be sure to eat before or as you're drinking. As we've seen, that helps alcohol exit the blood stream more quickly. For now, drink water. The more water you drink, the more you'll need to use the bathroom, which means you're eliminating waste and toxins, including alcohol, from your body. When all else fails, hit the sack. Time and sleep are truly the best cures for a hangover.

when to eat what

I wake up fine and get out the door, but after being at my desk a few minutes I'm ready for a snooze. What can I eat to keep my energy up through the morning?

A few things may be going on here. You don't mention food, and if you're simply drinking breakfast out of your coffee cup, that may be the root of your problem. Be sure to start the day with a breakfast containing carbs for energy (think fruits, oatmeal, whole grain breads, and cereals) and protein to keep you satisfied longer (think peanut butter, eggs, yogurt, milk). Plus, keep some of these healthy snacks on hand so you can munch on very small portions every hour or so:

- A handful of nuts
- Whole grain crackers
- A cheese stick
- Hummus and cut up veggies
- A glass of milk and a couple of graham crackers
- A piece of whole grain toast with peanut butter

With a carb and protein-balanced breakfast and snacks, you should be able to keep that 'get-up-and-go' feeling all morning.

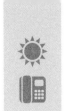

The vending machine at work is so enticing, especially on those long, late afternoons. Are there good choices I can make from it?

The vending machine doesn't need to be the diet and health saboteur it's made out to be. Don't get me wrong: Foods like fresh fruits and veggies and yogurt are certainly some of the healthier snacks out there, but decent choices can still be made from the vending machine.

The things I look for in a vending-machine snack are protein, fruit, and fiber. These components provide nutritional benefits, and the foods in which they're found don't tend to be loaded with unhealthy saturated fat and sodium. Protein takes longer to break down in the digestive system than carbohydrates. That means protein-filled foods stay in your stomach longer, and they keep you feeling fuller longer. Choosing snacks with protein, like nuts, will provide a longer-lasting feeling of satiety, which may be the difference between getting you safely to dinner or leaving you looking for even more munchies. Fiber also takes longer to break down in your digestive system. So fiber-rich foods like whole grain crackers and breads as well as popcorn can keep you feeling fuller longer.

Keeping those key foods or nutrients in mind, as I scan the giant window of vending-machine food, there are items that jump out at me, in no particular order:

- Nuts
- Light or low-fat microwave popcorn
- Whole grain chips
- Whole grain crackers (plain or with peanut butter)
- Crunchy granola bars
- Chocolate-covered peanuts
- Chocolate-covered raisins
- Fig bars

Whether you're craving sweet or savory, crunchy or chewy you should be able to find something to meet your needs.

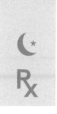

I tend to fall prey to the "I'm starving so I'm munching while I cook dinner" syndrome. What can I snack on that won't ruin my dinner?

This is a tough time of day, and that's usually due to the fact that it's been too long since lunch and now you're surrounded by food. Three to four hours is about the time it takes for a meal to mostly digest. As the food disappears, your insulin levels drop slightly, and hunger creeps in as a signal that your body is ready for its next meal. Unfortunately, for many of us that timing often coincides with getting home from work and making dinner. Prevention is the best solution. Add an afternoon snack to your day at the midpoint between your usual lunch-time and usual dinnertime. A simple, convenient snack you can make ahead is dried fruit and nuts. The fruit is full of simple carbohydrates, which will give you some quick energy to get you through the end of the day, while the protein-packed nuts will help prevent that sudden slump that often occurs after we eat quick-energy foods (translation: fruit or simple carbs) alone. In fact, nuts are full of healthy benefits. Walnuts specifically are a great source of omega-3 fatty acids in the diet. These fatty acids offer mega-benefits to your health, especially to your cardiovascular system. They can help lower levels of two substances: C-reactive protein and plaque adhesion molecules, which are both signs of inflammation in your arteries that can increase your risk of heart disease. In addition, the omega-3s can lower the chances that you'll develop artery-clogging clots by reducing the chances of platelets sticking together. Blood clots in the brain are responsible for strokes, while those in the heart cause heart attacks.

There are numerous combinations of fruits and nuts, but a few good ones include:

- Almonds and dried cherries
- Cashews and raisins
- Walnuts and dried blueberries

Combine these items in a big bowl in the evening or on a weekend and then measure out ¼-cup portions into resealable bags or bowls.

A second solution is to have some crudités as you prepare dinner. (Sure, I just mean veggie sticks, but doesn't crudités sound a bit fancier?) Pull out several sticks and chomp on them as you cook. This will make a dent in that hunger, it won't spoil your dinner, and it will provide you with an extra serving of veggies.

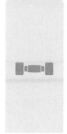

I'm training for a triathlon. I've heard that carb loading can cause weight gain. What can I eat leading up to a race that will give me the energy I need but help me lose weight, too?

Endurance events like triathlons and marathons do require carb loading to help maximize your body's ability to perform at its best for as long as possible. But there can be a price. Certainly, on the day of the race your body will be burning energy like there's no tomorrow, but in the days and weeks leading up to the race, you won't be using nearly as much energy. Still, you most likely require more food to sustain training, so the trick is finding that balance like you say of having just enough fuel, energy, carbs, and calories to keep you going but not so much that you can't lose weight (or that you even gain some).

The Institute of Medicine, the organization that determines the amount of every nutrient we need to eat each day to be healthy, recommends 130 grams of carbohydrates per day for all healthy Americans. One guide for endurance athletic events recommends about 4 grams of carbohydrate per pound as you prepare for a race. For a 170-pound person, that's about 680 grams of carbohydrates. And therein lies the problem. You need somewhere between 130 and 680 grams of carbohydrates per day to obtain the energy you need without going so overboard that you gain weight. Oh, and just a little FYI, those 680 grams of carbohydrates come in at about 2,700 calories. That's just carbs, not your protein or fat. Certainly not what you would call a weight-loss diet.

On the day before the event and on the day of the event itself, you must certainly ensure that your body has what it needs to do what you're asking of it. However, during your weeks and months of training, you can still make the adjustments necessary to lose the weight. During this time, break your diet down into two parts: your day-to-day healthy diet and your preworkout plan.

By themselves, losing weight and training for a triathlon are big commitments. Combined, they require a large chunk of motivation to carry through with what each task requires. To keep your day-to-day weight-loss goals in the forefront, determine your calorie needs (see Part 1). Then divide your daily calories into three meals, along with two or three snacks that include a variety of foods from each of the food groups. To learn how much food from each food group you should be eating, go to *www.mypyramid.gov*. Find the "I Want To" box and select "Get a personalized plan." Follow the steps to obtain a breakdown of the food groups created specifically for your needs.

Once you're eating well every day, it will be much easier to add in snacks before and after each workout. To improve your endurance and performance while you train, a good deal of research has shown you should eat carbohydrates between fifteen and sixty minutes before you plan to work out. This will give your muscles the energy they need to complete their task of running, biking, or swimming. The usual preworkout load in the majority of the studies was about 1 gram of carbohydrate per kilogram of body weight, along with 500 milliliters of water. So, between fifteen and sixty minutes before you plan to exercise, drink 2 cups of water or other fluid, along with 0.45 grams of carbohydrate for each pound you weigh. For a 150-pound person, that's about 68 grams of carbohydrates, and for a 200-pound person, it's about 91 grams of carbohydrates. You can experiment to find out what specific time works best for you to eat your snack, as well as if you should be getting all of your carbs from food or using some of those 2 cups of fluid to get some carbs in the way of a sports drink, juice, chocolate milk, or another type of carb-heavy drink. All packaged drinks will have a nutrition label informing you of the carb content per serving. There's also an assortment of packaged sports and energy bars and gels that also list carbohydrate content. Fruit also makes a great preworkout carb snack. One serving, which in most cases is a medium-sized piece of fruit or the equivalent, contains about 15 grams of carbohydrates. Whole grains can also be a good choice. By mixing and matching and doing some basic math, you should easily be able to find a variety of pre-workout snacks to get you through your exercise each day.

By eating this way, you're providing your body the extra calories and carbohydrates it needs when it needs them, rather than consuming these extras all day, every day. Remember, though, after your race is over you must continue to follow your day-to-day healthy-eating schedule, and keep in mind that your snacks don't need to be nearly as large as your pre-workout training snacks.

I'm going to a weekend brunch, but I usually get up early and I know I'll get hungry beforehand. What should I eat to tide me over?

Going to a late brunch on an empty stomach after being up for hours is a disaster waiting to happen. A smaller than usual breakfast at your usual breakfast time should fit the bill just fine. The one thing I wouldn't do is eat only fruit for your prebrunch breakfast. Fruit will fill you up for a time, but it digests quickly, and in terms of sugar levels, what goes up must come down. After that initial sense of fullness, you may find yourself even hungrier and walk into that brunch ready to eat everything in sight.

That being said, fruit can be a part of the solution. Pairing fruit with a nut butter such as an almond or peanut butter will both slow the digestion of the fruit and provide longer-lasting satisfaction from the protein and healthy fat. Nuts work in much the same way. Sliced peaches topped with slivered almonds are a delicious combination. An apple spread with cashew butter would be ideal as well. A low-fat dairy food such as yogurt or a reduced-fat cheese stick offers the same protein and fat the nuts do and could also pair well with fruit.

Of course, just a small serving of any of these ideas is what you need so you don't spoil your brunch. To keep calories in check, limit your serving to 1 ounce nuts, which is about 23 almonds, 28 peanuts, 8 to 10 walnuts, or 49 pistachios.

> **MAKE IT WORK FOR YOU**
>
> I'm always getting asked, "How can you eat nuts? They're so full of fat!" Nuts do contain a fair amount of fat, so go easy on your serving size. But they are full of beneficial fats that help prevent heart disease, and they offer protection from age-related diseases like Alzheimer's and more.

When I get sick, my healthy eating goes down the drain. As I start to feel better, I just eat whatever I want, and that's when the problems begin—I have to re-motivate myself to resume my healthy eating. How can I make the transition from sick eating to healthy eating without the junk in the middle?

It's a tough spot: You've felt miserable, so it's easy to tell yourself that you deserve some junk food after all you've been through. Well, ignore that little voice. To stay on track, simply use your sick foods as a basis to resume healthy eating again. Once you start to feel like you're ready to move beyond the broth-and-toast stage, bump up their nutrient quotient. Make sure the toast is whole grain, and top it with some peanut butter one day and maybe a fruit butter (like apple or pumpkin) the next day. To the broth, you can add leftover cooked veggies, low-sodium canned veggies, or some thawed frozen vegetables. And diced chicken or some drained and rinsed low-sodium canned beans will help you start to get more protein as your hunger grows. It's easy to expound on those meals little by little until you're back to your usual healthy-eating self.

You may have noticed I included both canned and frozen veggies in my suggestions here. Fresh vegetables seem to be considered by many to be the gold standard of vegetable nutrition, but you never know how long that produce sat on a truck or in a warehouse or even on the market shelves waiting to be bought and enjoyed by you. Canned and frozen vegetables, on the other hand, while often thought of as second class, are often packaged within hours of being harvested. And the packaging process seals in whatever nutrients they had at that moment in time—no deterioration or loss of vitamins beyond that point. This means that often the bag of frozen cauliflower or the can of green beans may very well contain more nutrients and be "fresher" than the fresh veggies in the produce department. I'm not saying to stop buying fresh veggies—not at all. If you buy local, there's little of the wait and transport time involved. All I'm saying is that since canned and frozen vegetables are less expensive and more convenient, there's no reason not to include them as part of your regular diet.

when to eat what

I've heard that potatoes, pasta, and bread are fattening and unhealthy, so I've stopped eating them. But I'm getting tired of just vegetables and meat, and I miss my sandwiches. What else can I eat that's not fattening?

It's true that those foods could cause you to gain weight, *but only if you eat too much of them.* In fact, ALL food can lead to weight gain if you eat too much of it. One of the problems many of us have with eating healthy and dieting is that we label foods as Good or Bad: something you *can* eat or something you *can't.* But that's just not the way it works. Labeling food as good or bad only sets you up for all kinds of problems. There's room for just about any food in a healthy diet. (Okay, so maybe not batter-dipped, deep-fried Twinkies or Snickers bars.) In my experience, when you label certain foods as bad and ban them, the food begins to seem even more desirable. You know the old saying: You want what you can't have. This often holds true when it comes to food. You swear to never eat chocolate again and you do great for a few days. Then, you see a chewy brownie or candy bar that looks especially good. Still you resist, but the urge keeps growing in your head until you can't take it and you eat all the chocolate you can find. Not real helpful when you're trying to lose weight.

Even if you're successful at cutting certain foods out of your diet, you can still end up in trouble because you may also be cutting out valuable nutrients—vitamins, minerals, and fiber found in that food. Not real helpful when you're trying to eat healthy. If you really need to use the labels good and bad, why not try using them to label serving sizes: A good serving of ice cream is ¼ or ½ cup; a bad serving of ice cream is a pint or a quart.

So, go ahead and enjoy your pasta, breads, and potatoes, but work on keeping your portions under control. A common trick I use is to pretend your plate is one of those divided ones that little kids use. Pretend the plate is divided into quarters. The lean protein portion of your meal should be no bigger than one of the quarters. Stacking food like a skyscraper doesn't count. The grain or starch portion of your meal should cover another quarter. The foods included in this category include potatoes, pasta, corn, peas, and rice. Go easy on the added fats and salt. Finally, fill the remaining section (half of the plate) with all kinds of vegetables—cooked or raw. This could be a combination of a crisp salad along with some cooked veggies, or it could be all cooked or all raw. It can be the same vegetable or an assortment of many. As with the starchy foods, go easy on the high-fat condiments. However, this is the section of your plate for which it's alright if the food overflows. These are low-calorie, high-fiber, high-nutrient foods. Fruits can also be included in this section, but due to fruit's higher calorie content, you'll want to limit the amount to about one serving.

A recent study in the *American Journal of Clinical Nutrition* showed how beneficial eating more fruits and vegetables is when trying to lose weight. Study participants were divided into two groups. One group followed a low-fat diet. The second group followed the same low-fat diet but also increased their intake of high-water-content foods like fruits and vegetables. After six months, those in the second group lost a third more weight than those who only cut their fat intake. After twelve months, the weight loss was still greater in the fruit-and-vegetable group. That group also reported feeling less hungry—a big bonus when trying to eat less and lose weight.

Here's another step you can take. When you eat these starchy foods, make sure you're maximizing the nutrient bang you get from them. When you eat a sandwich, use whole grain bread. Feel like some spaghetti? Use whole wheat. If the texture is a bit too tough, try overcooking it a bit. When preparing and eating potatoes, leave the skin on. These small changes will increase the nutrients, including fiber, in your food. As a result, you'll feel more satisfied from your meals and will be less likely to overeat.

when to eat what

I've heard I should drink green tea if I'm trying to lose weight. Will it help? How much should I drink?

Research has shown that tea is extremely beneficial to our health in a number of ways, not the least of which is weight loss. Recently, researchers in the Netherlands found that drinking green tea helped study participants burn more fat, lose less muscle, feel more satisfied and full, and lose weight. Polyphenols, which are substances found in many plants that both give them their bright colors and offer many health benefits to the human body, along with caffeine are believed to be responsible for these results. To achieve the results in the study, the participants consumed 270 milligrams catechins, a specific type of polyphenol found largely in tea, along with 150 milligrams of caffeine. All brands of tea vary slightly in their content, but you can find the appropriate amount of EGCG (the polyphenol found in green tea) and caffeine in about 2 to 3 cups of green tea.

One concern, however, is that not all the catechins in green tea may withstand the process of being digested. Another study looked at this and found that a simple addition to your tea will help you maximize your catechins absorption and, therefore, your possible weight loss. Simply adding milk (cow, rice, or soy) to your tea increased the available catechins from less than 20 percent to more than 50 percent. In the study, the amount of milk added was about half of the total tea amount. So, if you had 8 ounces of tea, you would add about ½ cup milk. Another option that brought the catechin availability up to as high as 75 percent was the inclusion of citrus juice. Using either lime, orange, or lemon juice in place of up to half of the water resulted in this increase.

MAKE IT WORK FOR YOU

The benefits of green tea go far beyond the scale. It has also been shown to be a soldier in the fight against heart disease. Research has shown that drinking green tea regularly can lower your risk of heart disease by lowering your LDL (bad blood cholesterol levels) as well as increasing your HDL (good cholesterol levels). In addition, it appears that green tea may play a role in cancer protection.

If you're going to be drinking this much green tea, you may find you want a little variety to prevent boredom. Just a couple of simple tricks can give you unlimited possibilities when it comes to making delicious green tea. For hot teas, simply add a couple tablespoons of a flavorful juice after brewing. Think blueberry, pomegranate, and other flavor-packed juices. If you want to add some variety to your iced green tea, brew your tea as usual (1 tea bag in 1 cup of hot water), chill it, and then serve it over ½ cup of your favorite frozen fruit. You could use raspberries, blackberries, or chopped melon just to name a few.

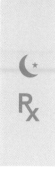

Most nights, after dinner, I find myself eating ice cream, cookies, chips, you name it, simply for lack of anything better to do, just out of habit. In one night I can easily eat a half a bag of chips or a pint of ice cream and I'm not even hungry. I know this isn't healthy, but what can I eat while vegging on the couch?

It sounds as though you're eating more out of boredom than anything else. To handle that, we have to look at this from more than one angle. First, since you know you grab these less-than-healthy, high-calorie foods in the evening, a good start would be to get them out of the house. It's one thing to have to get out of your comfy chair and walk all the way into the kitchen for a snack. But if you have to get out of that comfy chair, put on your shoes, get in the car, and drive to the store, you're much less likely to do it. I can hear your arguments now: "But my husband [or girlfriend, or kids, or roommate] eats those chips and cookies!" I have two responses to that: One, they don't need to be eating that much of those kinds of foods, either. Grabbing a single-serving bag of chips to go with a sandwich or going out for a special ice cream cone after dinner *once in a while* is a nice treat. Having 24-hour access to an array of fat-laden, sugar-filled, calorie-packed foods is a big reason this country has the overweight and obesity problems it does. Two, if they are grown adults and really want to have those foods around every day, ask them to buy them themselves and keep them somewhere you don't know about.

The second branch of the food part of this answer involves having foods around on which you can munch while watching your favorite television show. There are several foods that fit the bill, including:

- Air-popped or light microwave popcorn—you can eat as is, or mist with a couple of squirts of butter-flavored spray and sprinkle with your favorite seasonings, like cinnamon and sugar, chili powder, or Chinese 5-spice, to name a few
- Baked whole grain tortilla chips with salsa

- Frozen grapes or cherries
- Edamame
- Freeze-dried fruit or veggies
- Frozen fruit bars such as Edy's Fruit Bars
- Soy chips

The big rule with any snack, even healthy ones, is to never eat out of the box or bag. Serve out one portion, put the rest away, and then bring that one serving to the living room. It's much harder to overeat when you actually run out of food. Plus, when you see a limited quantity, it may cause you to eat more slowly, making a smaller portion last longer.

And finally, here's a non–food-related, but equally important, idea to consider. If you're simply eating out of boredom, giving either your hands, mouth, or both something to do will help prevent that. For instance, you're not likely to start chowing on potato chips when you're chewing gum. Plus a doctor at the Mayo Clinic found that you burn 11 calories an hour chewing. Sure it's not much, but if you add those 11 calories burned chewing to the calories you saved by avoiding unhealthy snacks, it can make a big difference. You can also find a hobby. If you're knitting or scrapbooking or even doing a crossword puzzle, your hands aren't free to put bite after bite of food in your mouth.

If you're eating healthy and exercising throughout the day, eliminating the calories from your nightly mindless munching may be all it takes to get you from where you are now to where you want to be as far as your weight is concerned.

I'm starving after my workout! How can I satisfy my hunger without negating all the hard work I just did?

Numerous studies, including one in the *Australian Journal of Science and Medicine in Sport,* have reported that what your body needs most after exercise is carbohydrates to replace glycogen stores lost during the workout as well as fluid and electrolytes lost from sweating.

What is glycogen? Glycogen is a form of glucose, or sugar, that is readily available when your body needs it for energy. Say you're working out and either you didn't eat much, or your body has already used up the sugar/energy you ate. Then your body must turn to glycogen stores in muscles and the liver to be able to continue exercising. When you're done exercising, it's important to replace those glycogen stores as quickly as possible so they will be available the next time you need them. The best types of carbohydrate in this situation are simple ones, ones that are broken down and used by your body quickly and easily. Fruit, any kind, and 100% fruit juice are the best for this, followed by simple grains such as white rice, pastas, cereals, or breads.

Whether you're simply glowing a little or the sweat is dripping off of you, you need to replace fluids and electrolytes. Electrolytes are minerals found in your body's fluid—blood, urine, sweat. They need to be kept balanced properly for various functions in your body to go off without a hitch. When you sweat, you're altering the levels of these substances. The most common are sodium, calcium, and potassium. Restoring the proper balance is not at all

MAKE IT WORK FOR YOU

Bananas are a great source of potassium in the diet. A very large study of almost 60,000 adults showed that the more potassium in the participants' diets, the less likely they were to have and die from cardiovascular disease. The same study showed that sodium intake had the opposite effect. High sodium intake was linked with a greater chance of having or dying from cardiovascular disease. Bananas, like all fruits, are very low in sodium and therefore make a delicious little heart-healthy snack.

difficult because all of these minerals are found in common foods and drinks, and you don't need high amounts of them.

So you've finished your workout and are raring to eat. You want to make a choice that keeps all of these factors in mind, without completely replacing the several hundred calories you just burned off. I'd recommend one of the more filling fruits, like a banana. It gives you something to bite into and chew versus some of the higher-water-content foods that, while refreshing, may not satisfy a ravenous appetite. To wash down that banana, grab a cup of 100% fruit juice for some fluid and quick electrolytes, then plain water to satisfy the remainder of your thirst. While the fruit juice contains much needed sugar and minerals, it also contains a good deal of calories. Overdoing it could easily negate a lot of that workout.

I've mentioned water and 100% fruit juice, but those sports drinks that seem to be a fixture at most gyms, health clubs, and YMCAs also contain electrolytes. Sports drinks, namely Gatorade, were first developed to be used by the University of Florida football team to help the players get through their grueling workouts in the hot Florida sun. They are a quick and easy way to replace everything athletes lose—glycogen, fluids, and electrolytes—all in one. And they do their job perfectly. However, if you've just completed a brisk twenty-minute walk around the block, you probably want to bypass the Gatorade. Sports drinks are ideal, and meant to be, for someone who is exercising more than an hour or less than an hour, but very intensely. You could also argue that they would benefit anyone doing hard manual labor as their job or for several hours as well. But everyone else who drinks them is just getting extra sugar, calories, and salt they probably don't need.

I don't like to cook when I get home from work. What can I prepare ahead of time?

In the hustle and bustle of the world in which we live, many important behaviors are often pushed aside because they seem to take too long. Sitting down and enjoying a healthy meal is one of those unfortunate casualties of the time crunch. But if healthy eating and losing weight are goals of yours, you may want to move sitting down to dinner back to the top of the priority list. A recent study found that people who actually sit down to eat dinner, preferably with friends or family, actually eat more fruits and vegetables, specifically the super-healthy dark green and orange veggies. Conversely, those who eat on the run consume more soft drinks, fast food, total fat, and saturated fat while at the same time eating less healthy foods.

You may not have much time to cook when dinnertime rolls around, but that doesn't mean you don't have time to cook a healthy dinner just the same. In these times of long work days, multiple jobs, family, and social obligations, many of us are ready to hit the sack when we get home, not the kitchen. But lazy and poor cooking and eating habits lead to bigger waistlines and decreasing health. Moving healthy eating up on your priority list is crucial, and so is figuring out when preparing a healthy dinner can fit into your day. There are a couple of ideas that could help you out. Neither one is mind blowing, but they can sure save you time at dinner.

MAKE IT WORK FOR YOU

Slow cookers or Crock-Pots work by cooking food at a low temperature for a longer period of time than usual. For this reason, healthy boneless, skinless chicken breasts, which cook very quickly, can often end up dried out when cooked in a slow cooker. But you can still reap the convenience of slow cookers while enjoying a yummy and healthy chicken dinner. There are two options. One, start with frozen skinless, boneless chicken breasts or raw whole, bone-in chicken breasts so the long cooking time doesn't overcook the meat. Two, use boneless, skinless chicken thighs instead. For a 3-ounce portion you will get a few more calories, but not enough to make a big difference once or twice a week.

The first thing you should do is prep ahead. When you get home from the grocery store, get as many of the foods as you can ready for cooking. Wash and chop vegetables; divide meat, chicken, or seafood into meal-sized packages; cut meat into pieces if necessary (you can then freeze the meat that won't be used in the next two days). It may add an extra half hour on to your shopping day, but the time will make up for itself tenfold on a hectic weeknight when all the prep work is done for dinner and you just need to mix and cook. Another time saver here is prepared foods. Now I know I've said that most prepared, processed foods are full of sodium, fat, and calories, and that's true for *most* of them. But there are several foods available that can give you the extra help you need without compromising your health or weight. These include:

- Precut fruits and veggies from the salad bar
- Frozen vegetables in steamer bags (corn, green beans, broccoli, cauliflower, carrots, and more)
- No-cook lasagna noodles (which turns lasagna into a one-pan dish that takes just a few minutes to assemble)
- 90-second microwaveable brown rice pouches such as Uncle Ben's (a minute and a half and you have a whole grain side dish)
- Low-sodium canned beans and vegetables

The other time saver may be a bit retro but is a huge helper in the kitchen: a slow cooker with a removable liner. For most recipes you just dump and cook; how much easier can cooking get? How great would it be to come home to the smells of a dinner that's been cooking nice and slow all day long? You may be thinking, "Well, that sounds great, but I barely have time in the morning to eat breakfast let alone cook dinner." Never fear. You can do all the measuring, mixing, and pouring the night before. Place everything in the slow cooker's removable liner, cover, and refrigerate overnight. All you do in the morning is remove the cover, pop the liner into the slow cooker's heating element, turn it on, and go. If your meal doesn't include a veggie or a starch, you will still need to cook

when to eat *what*

those to go along with your entrée. But that can almost be done in the time it takes to get into comfy clothes and get the table set.

There are countless slow cooker cookbooks out there, and many specialize in healthy recipes. You can also check out *http://blog.foodnetwork.com/healthyeats* or *http://allrecipes.com/recipes/everyday-cooking/vegetarian/slow-cooker/main .aspx* for some healthy slow-cooker recipes. If you find recipes you'd like to try that may not be so healthy, you can always make substitutions and adjustments to recipes. You can use lean meats, low-fat dairy products, low-sodium and low-fat cream soups and stocks, and you can always add more vegetables than the recipe calls for.

I've never been a fan of breakfast foods. What are some healthy foods I can eat for breakfast besides cereal and eggs and juice?

The only hard-and-fast rule for breakfast is just to eat it. And, as long as you include a variety of healthy foods, it doesn't matter exactly what makes up your breakfast. Think of some things you do like to eat and pair that with the idea of multiple food groups. A few I've come up with include:

- A ham and cheese sandwich on whole grain bread with some low-fat yogurt and a pear
- Leftovers from last night's dinner: 2–3 ounces lean meat, chicken, or fish; 1 cup of veggies; and ½ to ¾ cup of a whole grain or starch, such as brown rice, pasta, or potatoes
- 1 slice of veggie or cheese pizza paired with some grapes
- A peanut butter and jelly sandwich on whole grain bread with a glass of skim milk and a nectarine

All of these suggestions include servings from at least three different foods groups to give you a breakfast that is loaded with a variety of nutrients, including fiber, protein, calcium, vitamin C, vitamin E, and more.

If meat-based sandwiches are a big part of your go-to breakfast, knowing how to navigate the array of choices at the deli counter is key to keeping your health and weight in check. The deli has a wide variety of meats and cheeses, some of which can be a moderately regular part of a low-fat diet while

when to eat what

others should be much more limited. The low-fat choices include turkey breast, ham, roast beef, and chicken. In addition, most delis offer an assortment of flavors of chicken breast, including buffalo, lemon pepper, barbecue, and more, to give you all sorts of variety when it comes to making a yummy sandwich. On the other side of the fat scale are the ones you should avoid (or at least eat only once in a while). These include bologna, salami, liverwurst, corned beef, and pastrami.

Even if you're choosing a lean deli meat, sodium is still an issue. Most deli meats are extremely high in sodium and therefore may not be a wise choice for every day of the week. However, once or twice a week should be fine. You can also choose low -sodium deli meats whenever possible to help keep your sodium intake down.

I find that I'm not normally hungry in the morning. Is it okay to wait and have breakfast at work? If so, what are some convenient and easy breakfasts for the office that are healthy and can help keep me on my weight-loss plan?

I've heard this often. Between grogginess and a rush to get ready in the morning, for many people their appetite just hasn't kicked in yet. There's nothing wrong with waiting to eat breakfast for a couple of hours after you wake up; the most important thing is just that you eat it. There are plenty of options out there for breakfast desk-side dining. The complexity depends on what your place of business has for you to work with. Most places these days have at least a microwave and a fridge; some even have a toaster. And the back of a desk drawer can make a perfect mini pantry.

Ideal foods for a desk pantry include:

- Instant packets of oatmeal (plain is best)
- Assorted nuts to sprinkle on cereal, in oatmeal, or make a trail mix
- Small jar of peanut butter
- Assorted dried fruits to sprinkle on cereal, in oatmeal, or make a trail mix
- Small containers or bags with serving-size portions of whole grain cereals such as Kashi, Total, Cheerios, or Raisin Bran

Instant oatmeal packets are at the top of my office stash list because they, along with the microwaveable cups of oatmeal, make terrific nutrient-packed breakfast choices. Oats are full of vitamins and fiber while at the same time low in fat and sodium. Being able to toss an individual packet or cup into your purse or briefcase means you can easily have a healthy breakfast anywhere you go. But they aren't all equally as nutritious. One packet of plain instant oatmeal has just 100 calories, 80 milligrams of sodium, and no sugar. Simply choosing a flavored packet instead will add an extra 60 calories, almost 200 milligrams of sodium, and 13 grams of sugar. And opting for the microwaveable cups brings the calories up to 200 and the sugar to 17 grams (more than 4 teaspoons of

when to eat *what*

sugar). To maximize the nutrition and flavor without hindering your weight-loss measures, choose the plain packets and sprinkle 1 teaspoon of brown or white sugar on top. You can even stir in dried fruits and nuts for more flavor.

Don't forget to keep a small bowl and a spoon at work, too. If your office has a toaster, you can store a small loaf of whole grain bread or bring in a few slices to work in the morning to make toast. Keep some skim milk at work or bring some to work in a cooler each morning along with some fresh fruit.

There's also another side to this problem. I've found that a lot of people have conditioned themselves to skip breakfast for a variety of reasons—morning rush, trying to cut calories, not sure what's healthy. It's been so long since they've stopped in the morning each day to eat breakfast that now their body doesn't expect it and doesn't bother to say, "Hey, feed me!" That doesn't mean you still don't need breakfast. It's the first chance you get to feed your body's engine and start making some headway into your daily nutrient needs. In this case, I'd start with something small, and I'd try eating it a bit earlier each day, little by little. In other words, instead of waiting until you get to work to eat, try eating something on the way to work: a banana at the bus stop or a yogurt on the train. You can eventually work yourself up to having breakfast at home before you leave. Other good grab-and-go options are a fruit-and-grain bar, a few mini sandwiches made with peanut butter and whole grain crackers, and nuts mixed with dried fruit. All of these suggestions give you a good mix of energy-boosting carbs as well as protein, which takes longer to digest and therefore keeps you feeling fuller longer.

MAKE IT WORK FOR YOU

Oats are a terrific source of soluble fiber. The particular type of soluble fiber found in oats, beta glucan, has been shown in numerous studies to be an asset in protecting and improving cardiovascular health. Including oats in your diet helps lower your bad (LDL) cholesterol without lowering your good (HDL) cholesterol.

R_X I know that I should drink plenty of water each day. When is the best time to drink it, and how much do I need to drink?

When you are trying to lose weight, drinking water before a meal is a great trick. Multiple studies have been done on the subject, and the results of each are more promising than the last. The first showed that when participants drank 12 to 16 ounces of water about half an hour before a meal, they reported feeling more full at mealtime than those who had no water. This was followed up by a study in which the water drinkers again drank about 16 ounces half an hour before a meal and actually ate about 13 percent less food—about 75 calories—than those who did not drink water before a meal. If you do the math, three meals a day, seven days a week, you end up not eating the equivalent of about one pound every two weeks simply because you drank some water before your meal. Researchers saw this possibility, too, and decided to prove it. They did the same study except followed the participants for twelve weeks. Sure enough, those who drank the water while following a low-calorie diet lost 44 percent more weight than the ones who just followed the low-cal diet without drinking water before each meal.

But how much water does a person need? Well, that's a much trickier question. It's dependent on so many factors—not the least of which are weight, activity level, and the weather. The recommendation of eight to ten 8-ounce glasses a day has been around for a long time. The Institutes of Medicine, the organization that develops the Daily Recommended Intake (DRI) for all nutrients, recommends 3.7 liters per day for adult men and 2.7 liters per day for adult women. They also assume that about 20 percent of that water will come from high-water-content foods. So

MAKE IT WORK FOR YOU

Water does much more than help facilitate weight loss. It is necessary for your body to function properly. It carries nutrients to cells throughout the body and can help lubricate joints. Water aids in proper digestion of food and in the removal of waste and toxins from the body, which leads to clearer, brighter-looking skin.

when to eat what

when you do all the math, it works out to be about 8½ cups for women and 12½ cups for men.

Another guideline is 1 ounce per kilogram of your ideal body weight. (To convert pounds to kilograms, just divide by 2.2.) For example, if your healthy weight is 150 pounds, that would be about 68 kilograms, which means you need 68 ounces of water (about eight and a half 8-ounce glasses). Whichever recommendation you choose to follow, they are all fairly similar, and they are certainly not going to put you at risk for either consuming too little or too much water.

You need the fluid, yes, but it's perfectly fine—and in fact, expected—to get some of it from a juicy piece of watermelon or a handful of grapes or from any other food with a high water content. But when it comes to other beverages counting as your fluid intake, you need to give it a bit more thought. For a long time, the word on the street was not to count coffee and tea and other caffein-ated beverages as part of your fluid intake. You're drinking fluids to hydrate yourself, so common sense would say that the fluids that dehydrate you (coffee, etc.) shouldn't really count. However, research has shown that for people who drink beverages containing caffeine *on a regular basis*, there appears to be no additional loss of fluids following the caffeine ingestion. Bottom line: if you usually drink a cup or two of coffee or a few cups of tea per day, go ahead and check them off as part of your daily fluid count.

Alternatively, if you're trying to lose weight, then 8 to 10 cups of sugar-filled, calorie-packed drinks such as sodas, sugar-sweetened teas or lemonades, and other fruit drinks probably isn't the best idea. So again, if you want one on occa-sion, great, but don't count it as part of your daily fluid.

Skim milk and 100% fruit juice are certainly loaded with nutrients and aren't terribly high in calories, but again, too much of a good thing isn't always a good thing. Go ahead and count the milk and juice as part of your daily fluids, but don't strive to get all eight to ten glasses from them. For the purpose of calorie reduction, your best bet once you've counted two or three glasses of milk and a glass of juice is to just enjoy the five or six remaining glasses as simple, refresh-ing water.

Dieting gives me a headache in the afternoon! What can I eat to stave off my headaches and keep my diet on track?

Before we look at what you can eat to stave off your headaches, it's helpful to take a look at what might be causing them in the first place. Nutritionally speaking, there are a couple of things that could be giving you headaches, and there are some pretty simple fixes. However, if you don't see improvement with these suggestions, I'd recommend getting yourself checked out by your health care provider to rule out any more troubling issues.

Often, being dehydrated can lead to headaches. Food seems to take top billing, especially when trying to lose weight—what should I eat, what shouldn't I eat, how much should I eat, when should I eat it—and beverages and what and how much to drink don't really get the attention they deserve and need to maintain your body's health. Ensuring that you're drinking enough water may be all you need to get rid of those headaches and, as we've seen, give your diet a boost.

In a 2008 study, researchers found that when study participants drank 4 cups of water a day, in addition to following a weight-loss diet, they lost an additional 5 pounds a year. That's above and beyond the weight lost from the diet alone. In addition, study participants also saw a decrease in their waistline and body-fat percentage. The scientists attribute this weight loss and other changes to the idea that drinking that amount of water actually causes your body to burn more calories.

Another possible cause of afternoon headaches is hypoglycemia—when the levels of sugar in your blood get too low—which may present itself through other symptoms such as sweating, dizziness, and intense hunger. Eating too little, a common practice of dieters, is one possible cause of this. To counteract possible hypoglycemia, make sure that you're eating enough food. Eat three meals a day as well as small snacks between meals. And, while you need lean protein and healthy fats as part of a balanced diet, be sure you're not skimping on carbohydrates. There are popular diets around that recommend banning carbohydrates, but in fact, carbohydrates are your body's main source of fuel and they provide the most readily available energy your body has to function every day. Restricting your carbohydrate intake too severely may certainly lead to low blood sugar and annoying headaches. But the problems don't stop there.

When your body doesn't have the sugar it needs, it starts breaking down muscle for fuel. That's the last thing you want to happen because, as we've noted, the more muscle you have, the more calories you burn. Once your body begins to break down muscle for energy, you must eat fewer calories to prevent weight gain, and you must work that much harder to lose weight. Not a pretty picture.

When it comes to carbohydrates, you definitely need them as part of a healthy diet. At the same time, you want to choose those that are more complex and full of nutrients. Select whole grain breads and cereals versus cakes and pastries made with sugar and refined (white) flour. Fruits versus candy. You get the picture. But what exactly are whole grains? And what's the difference between whole grains and fiber? It can be confusing. While the two are related, they are not the same thing. Fiber is the indigestible part of the plant foods we eat. It's found in fruits, vegetables, and grains. There are different types of fiber, and they help our digestive system run more smoothly, protect us from heart disease, and more.

Whole grains, on the other hand, contain fiber, along with an assortment of vitamins. A whole grain is exactly what it says it is—a "whole" grain. When wheat and other grains are refined, two of the edible portions, the bran and the germ, are removed. These parts are where the majority of the nutrients are found in grains. By replacing your refined grains with whole grains, you'll eat more nutrients, including fiber, vitamin E, and B vitamins. Many food packages now come with a stamp letting you know if a food is considered a whole grain food. According to the FDA, a food must have been made with at least 51 percent of a whole grain ingredient to be legally called a whole grain food. You can also look at the ingredient list on food packages. You want a whole grain to be at least one of the first few ingredients. Examples of whole grains are wheat, barley, brown rice, bulgur, corn, oats, quinoa, and rye. Another clue is to look for the word *whole* in front of one of the first few ingredients.

To sum up, to try to get rid of your headaches while making sure you keep to your diet, be sure to drink the proper amount of fluids every day. Don't skip meals, and in fact, if you're going longer than three to four hours between meals, plan a small snack. Follow these guidelines, and hopefully your headaches will be a thing of the past.

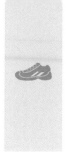

I belong to a variety of social organizations, and it seems like every time I turn around, there's another potluck to go to. What is a healthy contribution to take to a potluck so I can have something to choose for my dinner but not blow my diet once a week?

Potluck dinners, covered dish suppers, progressive dinners, or whatever else you may call them are usually made up of an evening full of friends, fun, and delicious food that is often packed full of cheese, butter, and an assortment of other yummy but high-fat ingredients. If you take part in one once in a blue moon, your donation as well as your dinner selection probably aren't that significant. However, if your social calendar is chock full, you need a game plan for taking part in all of the food-based fun while keeping your waistline and health where you want it. Here's a course-by-course list of suggestions for what to bring or how to change some of your already favorite dishes.

MAKE IT WORK FOR YOU

The health benefits of walnuts are plenty. Studies have shown that people who include walnuts in their diet are less susceptible to cardiovascular events such as heart attacks and strokes. Italian researchers have found that as little as four walnuts a day can raise the levels of healthy fatty acids in the blood.

- **First course or appetizers:** Often, these are fried little tidbits of some sort of meat or creamy, cheesy fillings overflowing from buttery little cups of pastry. Why not add some fruit to the mix of choices? A simple, light fruit salad will provide fiber and water, both of which can help fill you up so you'll eat less of the more calorie-heavy dishes. Other possibilities include melon wrapped in thin slices of prosciutto or berry kabobs.
- **Salads:** Here's an opportunity to get some vegetables into the meal in place of the usual mayonnaise- or sour cream–based salads such as macaroni, potato, and coleslaw. A baby spinach and strawberry salad topped with chopped walnuts is bursting with antioxidant power, not to mention

extremely low calories. Dress it simply with a basic vinaigrette and you've got the easiest potluck dish around. If you're really looking for one of those creamy salads, then a few simple tweaks can improve their nutrition profile. Instead of using full-fat mayo or sour cream, substitute a mixture of reduced-fat mayo or sour cream and fat-free plain yogurt as your base. In addition, you can shred or chop lots of extra veggies to mix in, such as carrots, zucchini, cucumber, broccoli, and more.

- **Sides:** This is where you usually find all those cheesy, creamy potato dishes. Why not give sweet potatoes a whirl? With more than a day's worth of vitamin A, a good dose of potassium, and barely a trace of fat, they're an ideal basis for a healthy side dish. Simply mash some cooked sweet potatoes with a touch of butter and brown sugar, some cinnamon, and a splash of orange juice, and you've got a colorful side dish fit for a king—a healthy king, at least. You could also take a favorite rice dish, such as a pilaf filled with slivered almonds. Just use brown rice in place of the white for a more filling dish that's packed with fiber and vitamins.

- **Entrées:** These tend to be a bit more of a challenge. Depending on where you live, commonplace entrées are often fried chicken, sausage and peppers, barbecued ribs, or ooey-gooey lasagna. Chicken or even a bean-based dish are probably your best bets for a healthy entrée. A hearty bean chili is great for a winter gathering, while seasoned, grilled, boneless, skinless chicken breasts work well in the summer. A simple grilled chicken is good hot or cold and can be eaten as is or on a sandwich. A big pan of barbecued pulled pork or chicken is a nice option, too. You can even make the lasagna work. Simply use reduced-fat cheeses and replace the sausage with zucchini or spinach for an extra nutrient kick.

- **Desserts:** Fudgy brownies, multicolored cupcakes, and creamy, chocolaty, layered desserts are usually on every potluck dessert table. And, if you've chosen a well-balanced, nutritious meal, there's certainly nothing wrong with having a small piece of a rich dessert to finish the meal. But there are also several dishes you could bring to offer a lighter dessert choice. A simple dark chocolate fondue is always popular. Bring fruit slices and angel food cake

when to eat what

cubes as your dippers. Speaking of angel food cake, use it to make a light and fruity trifle. Simply layer cubes of angel food cake with low-fat vanilla pudding, a light whipped topping, and sliced strawberries and kiwi.

Perhaps you have a few favorite recipes you hate to part with while you're trying to whittle your waistline. I've got good news for you. These favorite dishes do not have to be a casualty of losing weight. There are many simple substitutions you can incorporate as you cook to lower the fat and calorie content of your favorite foods but still retain the flavors you long for. Maybe you've already thought about substituting ingredients but you aren't sure how the recipe will come out. Here are a few easy ingredient substitutions that should still result in recipe success:

Instead of this . . .	Try this . . .
Condensed cream soups	Reduced-fat-and-sodium cream soups
Sour cream	Reduced-fat sour cream or nonfat plain yogurt
Whole milk	Skim or 1% milk
Evaporated milk	Skim evaporated milk
Cream or half-and-half	Fat-free half-and-half
Heavy cream	Skim evaporated milk
Cheese	Reduced-fat cheese
Chicken thighs or legs	Boneless, skinless chicken breast (will need to reduce cooking time if recipe calls for bone-in chicken)
Cream cheese	Reduced-fat cream cheese
Oil in baking	Cut the amount down by ¼ to ⅓
Butter or shortening in baking	Nonfat plain yogurt, fat-free sour cream, or replace half with well-mashed ripe avocado
1 cup chocolate chips	½ cup mini chocolate chips

There are days when my errands have me out the door from 9:00 A.M. until mid-afternoon. I usually end up skipping lunch or grabbing a bite at the closest fast-food drive-through. What else can I do on these days?

Pretend you're back at school and pack a lunch, or at the very least, pack a hearty snack. You'll not only save on fat and calories, but you'll also save some much-needed time and money. You don't have to pack anything fancy, just something to prevent a fast- food run a couple times a week.

You should try to go no longer than three to four hours without eating to help prevent yourself from getting overly hungry and then overeating. So having a healthy lunch with you is a great plan to possibly help prevent unnecessary weight gain or to make weight loss a bit easier. I'd start with getting a small cooler and an ice pack. There's nothing worse than a hot, cold lunch. This will also help keep perishable food safe for a few hours. When thinking about packed lunches, especially something that will be eaten in a car, start with a sandwich, veggies, drink, and fruit. This way you know you're covering all the bases, and you can then tackle each category one by one. It may sound like this basic lunch could be pretty boring over and over again, but it's not like you're eating it day after day. Plus, there's a ton of room for creativity within each group. If you're not sure what to pack, choose one option from each category here:

- **Sandwiches:** For fillings, there's the old standby, PB & J, but you can vary that with different nut butters, all-fruit spreads, fruit butters, and more. If deli meats are more your style, go with low-sodium ham, turkey, chicken, or roast beef, which are the leanest options. The choices don't end there: you can get honey ham, Italian roast beef, buffalo chicken, and the list goes on. Then for the bread—sliced bread, pitas, tortillas, lavash bread, English muffins, and more (all whole grain, of course).
- **Vegetables:** Be sure you always have a variety of veggies you like to eat raw on hand. Beyond just the basic baby carrots, think cucumber, celery, cherry tomatoes, red or green bell peppers, cauliflower, broccoli, and more. Any of

these offer a nice little crunch with or without a small amount of reduced-fat dip.

- **Drinks:** This is probably the most limited of the groups. You want a drink that's nutritionally beneficial but does not overload you with calories. Fill a small Thermos or leak-proof cup with 1 cup of skim or 1% milk or 1 cup of 100% juice, or even just bring some icy cold water.

- **Fruits:** Fruit is a sweet ending to any meal. Almost any kind of fruit can be tossed, gently of course, into a lunch bag. Go ahead and explore the produce aisle to get whatever is currently in season. This is nature's way of adding variety to your diet: fall apples; winter clementines and pomegranates; spring and summer's bountiful array of berries, peaches, nectarines, apricots, plums, and more. And there are always the old standbys of bananas and grapes. Don't forget dried fruit, either. This category used to be limited to raisins, plums (aka prunes), and dates, but now you can find dried cranberries, blueberries, cherries, apricots, apples, and more. Canned fruit packed in juice vs. syrup is an option, too. One last note: if you bring 100% fruit juice as your drink, then pack a container of low-fat yogurt in place of fruit. This way you're still getting 1 fruit serving and 1 dairy, instead of 2 fruits and no dairy.

MAKE IT WORK FOR YOU

Think beyond peanut butter. Try some different nut butters, such as almond, cashew, or soy nut. You might think eating fatty foods like nuts and nut butters would cause weight gain, but research says otherwise. In a study on almonds, researchers found that a daily serving didn't cause weight gain. When participants ate the nuts, they naturally modified their intake of other foods the rest of the day to make up for the fat and calories in the nuts. Plus, nuts contain healthy fats that are beneficial in disease protection and prevention, especially as far as cardiovascular health is concerned.

When you break it down like this, you can see how taking a few extra minutes in the morning, or even the night before, to pack a lunch is really pretty easy and well worth the calorie, fat, time, and money savings.

After work, it's all I can do to get to the couch for a nap, but then I wake up starving and chow down on whatever I can find. What can I eat to change this cycle?

Fatigue from work leaves a lot of people ready to crash. And there's nothing wrong with that, as long as it doesn't interfere with your healthy-eating habits. However, if this is your usual routine, I'd recommend a snack on the way home from work. Just get a little something in your stomach so that when you wake up from your nap you're not starving. This will give you time to prepare a healthy dinner when you wake up instead of eating anything and everything in sight. As it stands, your current routine leaves you filling up on a random mix of whatever foods are quick and easy and then you're not hungry for dinner.

In addition, perhaps you're not eating adequately through the day and are suffering the effects. Make sure you're eating an adequate lunch; you can check out the menus in the back of the book from some simple, healthy ideas. In addition, an afternoon snack would be beneficial in this situation.

Either just before you leave for work or on the way home if you're not driving, have a moderate-sized snack. Refer to the two-week menu in Part 3 for several snack examples. It can be anything, really. Just avoid something that's mostly or all simple carbohydrates; such a snack would be completely digested by the time you woke up from your nap, and you'd be no better off than you were before. Foods and drinks like candy, pastries, cookies, soda, sweetened coffee or tea drinks, and even fruit if it's all by itself could have this effect. Also avoid other empty-calorie foods that contribute nothing to your diet but fat or salt. These are all right once in a while as part of a healthy diet, but as a daily snack, they're a big waste of calories. And if you're trying to keep your calorie intake under control to lose weight, they aren't a wise choice. These include potato chips, cheese puffs, French fries, and other foods along those lines.

So what does that leave? Plenty. You want to avoid fruit by itself, but there's nothing wrong with having some fruit together with a fiber- or protein-rich food such as reduced-fat cheese, nuts, peanut butter, whole grain crackers, edamame, or air-popped or light microwave popcorn. A half of a small sandwich could also be a good postwork/prenap snack as well. You see, there are a great many foods and food combinations that will serve your purposes perfectly by letting you enjoy your much-needed rest but also allowing you to wake up able to prepare and enjoy a healthy meal.

There's also the possibility that you may be feeling the need to crash because of the coffee you drank to keep you alert at work. Do you spend your day continually refilling your coffee cup? If so, that lull you feel once you get home may actually just be your body's response to its first caffeine-free time of the day. Caffeine has been shown to negatively affect sleep. In fact, a recent study from Hong Kong showed that drinking only decaf coffee for one whole day improved participants' sleep: they slept longer, slept more soundly, and fell asleep easier. Furthermore, other research has shown that dependence on caffeine can lead to an increase in daytime sleepiness. Make sure you're getting adequate sleep at night and eating appropriately throughout the day. Then, try weaning yourself off of the caffeine, or at least limit your coffee drinking to before lunch. This will allow you to get your day going with an extra jolt, but you'll also be training your body to learn to live life more naturally without a constant supply of caffeine.

And, last but not least, while it may sound counterintuitive to increase your activity level when you're tired, it's actually a great idea. Researchers at the University of Georgia found that people who began exercising regularly felt more energized and less tired than people who continued to follow a more sedentary lifestyle. Sure, it may be hard at first to force yourself to exercise when you feel so tired, but in the long run it'll be well worth it. Add a brisk fifteen-minute walk to your day either in the morning, at lunchtime, or at the end of your work day—really, wherever it fits into your day the easiest. Gradually work up to a half hour. Not only will the increased activity help you feel more energetic and alert, it can also help you lose weight and be fitter.

two-week meal plan

Part 1 discussed a few of the basics of eating healthy. Now it's time to put those guidelines into action and get started on your new nutritious path. First, you'll find a two-week meal plan full of delicious meals and snacks to get you through the day energized and satisfied. This is followed by simple modifications you can make to the meal plan if your usual routine or needs don't quite mesh with the menu.

As you scan through the meal plan, you'll notice that some meals or snacks are as simple as grabbing a couple items. Others require a few minutes of putting ingredients together or heating something up. Still others are a bit more elaborate. Never fear—recipes are here. For those items that require more specific cooking instructions, you'll find recipes at the end of this section of the book. Don't you dare shy away from them. The recipes are all very simple, and they only include foods found in your regular grocery store, if not your kitchen.

Each day provides around 1,800 calories worth of energy. If you need much more or less, see the modifications later in the book. Those calories are broken down into about 20 percent protein, 50 percent carbohydrate, and 30 percent fat. In addition, each day provides you with at least 25 grams of fiber and 1,000 milligrams of calcium, as well as no more than about 2,300 milligrams of sodium. You'll also notice that each day includes two snacks. Enjoy them wherever they fit best in your day. If you have an early breakfast and a late lunch, a midmorning snack may be just what you need.

As you go through the meal plan, remember that you need to have your food the way you like it. To me, a big part of healthy eating is enjoying what you're eating. The menu is not a hard-and-fast rule of what you have to eat. It's merely a suggestion to help get you started. You can follow it to the letter, or you can change it up to suit your tastes.

For example, if a banana is listed but you're more in the mood for a pear, by all means have a pear. Never been a fan of broccoli? Then go ahead and have some carrots or spinach. Of course, that being said, substituting a super-deluxe, fast-food burger for a turkey sandwich or a king-size candy bar for some yogurt won't give you quite the same results. But read on, and bon appetite!

two-week meal plan

DAILY NUTRITIONAL TOTALS

Calories: 1,684

Protein: 100 grams

Carbohydrates: 237 grams

Fiber: 27 grams

Total Fat: 39 grams

Saturated Fat: 12 grams

Sodium: 2,733 milligrams

Breakfast

Southwest Scramble (page 186)

1 slice whole grain toast with ½ teaspoon spreadable/tub margarine

1 peach

Lunch

Ham Roll Up (page 186)

1 cup skim milk

1 cup seedless grapes

½ medium cucumber (sliced)

DAILY NUTRITIONAL TOTALS

Calories: 1,546

Protein: 79 grams

Carbohydrates: 255 grams

Fiber: 39 grams

Total Fat: 29 grams

Saturated Fat: 7 grams

Sodium: 1,667 milligrams

Breakfast

Blueberry Cobbler Oatmeal (page 188)

Lunch

Crunchy Tuna Salad (page 188)

6 whole wheat crackers

1 cup skim milk

1 cup baby carrots

1 medium apple

DAILY NUTRITIONAL TOTALS

Calories: 1,699

Protein: 73 grams

Carbohydrates: 232 grams

Fiber: 30 grams

Total Fat: 58 grams

Saturated Fat: 18 grams

Sodium: 2,456 milligrams

Breakfast

2 whole grain frozen waffles topped with 1½ tablespoons Nutella

1 small banana (sliced)

1 cup skim milk

Lunch

Quick Mexican Pizza (page 189)

¾ cup diced cantaloupe

1 cup skim milk

two-week meal plan

Dinner

Italian Meatloaf (page 187)

1 medium baked potato with 1 teaspoon spreadable/tub margarine, 1 teaspoon reduced-fat sour cream, and a sprinkle of fresh chopped or dried chives

1 cup cooked carrots with ½ teaspoon spreadable/tub margarine

1 cup skim milk

Snack #1

¾ cup fat-free vanilla yogurt mixed with ⅓ cup blueberries and 1 tablespoon slivered almonds

Snack #2

1 ounce unsalted pretzels with ½ cup salsa

Day 1

Dinner

Super Easy Spaghetti: 1 cup cooked whole wheat pasta topped with ¾ cup low-sodium marinara/spaghetti sauce

1 cup tossed salad (lettuce, tomato, cucumber, red onion) topped with 1 tablespoon reduced-fat salad dressing

1 cup skim milk

Snack #1

12 medium strawberries with 1 chocolate fat-free pudding cup

Snack #2

1 medium pear with 1 ounce reduced-fat Cheddar cheese

Day 2

Dinner

Really Big Salad (page 190)

1 cup skim milk

Snack #1

¼ cup hummus with 6 whole wheat crackers

Snack #2

Trail Mix: 2 tablespoons dried fruit, 1 tablespoon nuts, and ¼ cup unsweetened cereal (like Crispix)

Day 3

Day 4

DAILY NUTRITIONAL TOTALS

Calories: 1,740

Protein: 80 grams

Carbohydrates: 196 grams

Fiber: 24 grams

Total Fat: 78 grams

Saturated Fat: 18 grams

Sodium: 2,176 milligrams

Breakfast

Breakfast Banana Split
(page 190)

Lunch

1 regular fast-food
cheeseburger

1 garden salad with
1 tablespoon reduced-fat
salad dressing

1 medium apple

Day 5

DAILY NUTRITIONAL TOTALS

Calories: 1,600

Protein: 74 grams

Carbohydrates: 230 grams

Fiber: 25 grams

Total Fat: 49 grams

Saturated Fat: 9 grams

Sodium: 1,928 milligrams

Breakfast

1½ cup whole grain cereal
(such as Cheerios or Life)
with 1 cup skim milk,
2 tablespoons walnuts,
and 1 tablespoon dried
cranberries

Lunch

1½ cups reduced-sodium
vegetable soup (such as
Progresso)

6 low-sodium saltine
crackers

1 cup skim milk, 1 medium
plum

Day 6

DAILY NUTRITIONAL TOTALS

Calories: 1,686

Protein: 109 grams

Carbohydrates: 213 grams

Fiber: 35 grams

Total Fat: 51 grams

Saturated Fat: 17 grams

Sodium: 3,214 milligrams

Breakfast

Cottage cheese parfait
(1 cup 1% fat, low-sodium
cottage cheese layered
with ½ cup blueberries)

1 whole grain English
muffin topped with
1 teaspoon tub/spreadable
margarine

Lunch

Salmon-Topped Salad
(page 194)

1 small (4") whole wheat
pita

½ cup raspberries mixed
into ¾ cup fat-free vanilla
or plain yogurt

Dinner

Grilled Salmon (page 191)

1 cup steamed green beans topped with
¼ teaspoon tub/spreadable margarine
and a dash of salt-free garlic-and-herb
seasoning

1 cup Lemon-Infused Couscous (page 191)

Snack #1

1 wedge The
Laughing Cow
Light cheese with
5 whole wheat
crackers

Snack #2

3 tablespoons
pistachios

Day 4

Dinner

Pan-Fried Italian Chicken (page 192)

Roasted Red Potatoes and Broccoli
(page 193)

Snack #1

1 medium
banana dipped
in 1 tablespoon
melted
semisweet
chocolate chips

Snack #2

3 cups Cinnamon
Popcorn
(page 194)

Day 5

Dinner

Takeout pizza (2 slices cheese or veggie-
topped thin-crust pizza)

1 cup mixed greens salad with
1 tablespoon reduced-fat salad dressing

Snack #1

1 (3-ounce)
toasted 100%
whole wheat
bagel topped
with 1 teaspoon
all-fruit spread

¾ cup skim milk

Snack #2

1 medium green
pepper, sliced,
dipped into ⅓
cup hummus

Day 6

two-week meal plan

Day 7

DAILY NUTRITIONAL TOTALS

Calories: 1,698

Protein: 94 grams

Carbohydrates: 258 grams

Fiber: 24 grams

Total Fat: 35 grams

Saturated Fat: 6 grams

Sodium: 1,767 milligrams

Breakfast

Apple Burrito (page 195)

1 cup skim milk

Lunch

Turkey Pita (page 195)

6 ounces low-fat yogurt

1 cup seedless grapes

Day 8

DAILY NUTRITIONAL TOTALS

Calories: 1,690

Protein: 86 grams

Carbohydrates: 236 grams

Fiber: 30 grams

Total Fat: 57 grams

Saturated Fat: 17 grams

Sodium: 2,088 milligrams

Breakfast

Sunshine Smoothie
(page 197)

2 slices 100% whole wheat toast with ½ teaspoon tub/spreadable margarine

Lunch

Nut-n-Honey Sandwich
(page 197)

1 cup skim milk

1 medium nectarine

Day 9

DAILY NUTRITIONAL TOTALS

Calories: 1,604

Protein: 86 grams

Carbohydrates: 199 grams

Fiber: 39 grams

Total Fat: 60 grams

Saturated Fat: 13 grams

Sodium: 1,497 milligrams

Breakfast

2 slices 100% whole grain toast topped with 1 teaspoon honey

½ cup fat-free vanilla yogurt with ½ cup sliced strawberries

Lunch

California Egg Salad Sandwich (page 198)

1 cup skim milk

½ medium cucumber cut into sticks

1 medium peach

when to eat *what*

two-week meal plan

Dinner

Soft Turkey Tacos (page 196)

¾ cup corn

Snack #1

6 ounces plain or vanilla nonfat yogurt with ½ cup sliced strawberries

Snack #2

2 tablespoons almonds mixed with 2 tablespoons raisins

Dinner

Ham and Sweet Potato Skillet (page 198)

1 cup skim milk

Snack #1

½ cup edamame with 1 ounce reduced-fat Cheddar cheese

Snack #2

3 chocolate candy kisses with 2 tablespoons peanuts

Dinner

Chicken Scampi (page 199)

¾ cup cooked whole wheat pasta

1 cup skim milk

Snack #1

1 cup baby carrots with 1½ tablespoons peanut butter

Snack #2

1 ounce pistachios

DAILY NUTRITIONAL TOTALS

Calories: 1,661

Protein: 78 grams

Carbohydrates: 265 grams

Fiber: 42 grams

Total Fat: 44 grams

Saturated Fat: 10 grams

Sodium: 1,772 milligrams

Breakfast

Breakfast Sandwich
(page 199)

1 cup skim milk

1 medium orange

Lunch

Crab Melt (page 200)

1 cup skim milk

1 cup diced melon

DAILY NUTRITIONAL TOTALS

Calories: 1,648

Protein: 83 grams

Carbohydrates: 260 grams

Fiber: 36 grams

Total Fat: 39 grams

Saturated Fat: 7 grams

Sodium: 2,162 milligrams

Breakfast

Rum Raisin Oatmeal
(page 201)

Lunch

English Muffin Pizza
(page 201)

¾ cup cucumber sticks with
1 tablespoon reduced-fat
veggie dip or dressing

¾ cup fat-free vanilla
or plain yogurt mixed
with ½ cup chopped
strawberries

DAILY NUTRITIONAL TOTALS

Calories: 1,674

Protein: 119 grams

Carbohydrates: 214 grams

Fiber: 29 grams

Total Fat: 38 grams

Saturated Fat: 10 grams

Sodium: 2,256 milligrams

Breakfast

¾ cup reduced-fat cottage
cheese with ½ cup
chopped pineapple

2 slices whole grain toast
topped with 1 teaspoon
tub/spreadable margarine

Lunch

1 6", fast-food, oven-roasted
chicken sub sandwich
(perhaps from Subway)

1 (1-ounce) bag Baked!
Lay's

1 (2-ounce) bag apple
slices

1 (12-ounce) container low-
fat milk

when to eat what

two-week meal plan

Dinner

Rice and Beans (page 200)

1 cup mixed greens salad with
1 tablespoon reduced-fat salad dressing

Snack #1

Trail Mix:
2 tablespoons dried fruit,
1 tablespoon nuts, and ¼ cup unsweetened cereal (like Crispix)

Snack #2

⅓ cup Slow Churned/reduced-fat vanilla ice cream sandwiched between 2 (2½" square) chocolate graham crackers

Day 10

Dinner

Thai Shrimp Noodles (page 202)

1 cup skim milk

Snack #1

1 ounce baked tortilla chips with ¼ cup salsa

Snack #2

3 cups Spicy Popcorn (page 203)

Day 11

Dinner

Grilled Chicken (page 202)

1 medium baked sweet potato with ¼ teaspoon cinnamon

1 cup steamed broccoli with ½ teaspoon tub/spreadable margarine

1 cup skim milk

Snack #1

½ medium red pepper sliced

½ cup baby carrots

⅓ cup hummus for dipping

Snack #2

2 oatmeal raisin cookies

1 cup skim milk

Day 12

two-week meal plan

Day 13

DAILY NUTRITIONAL TOTALS

Calories: 1,665
Protein: 102 grams
Carbohydrates: 226 grams
Fiber: 40 grams
Total Fat: 52 grams
Saturated Fat: 17 grams
Sodium: 3,926 milligrams

Breakfast

1 cup whole grain cereal (such as crispy brown rice cereal) with ¾ cup skim milk topped with ½ medium banana, sliced

Lunch

Roast Beef Sandwich (page 203)

1 cup skim milk

1 medium orange

¼ red bell pepper, sliced

Day 14

DAILY NUTRITIONAL TOTALS

Calories: 1,705
Protein: 89 grams
Carbohydrates: 269 grams
Fiber: 43 grams
Total Fat: 46 grams
Saturated Fat: 11 grams
Sodium: 2,067 milligrams

Breakfast

2 slices whole grain toast with 2 teaspoons apple butter

1 cup skim milk

½ medium banana

Lunch

PB&J (1 tablespoon peanut butter and 1 teaspoon all-fruit spread on 2 slices whole grain bread)

1 medium apple

1 cup skim milk

when to eat *what*

Dinner

Family-style restaurant's grilled shrimp and island rice (perhaps from Applebees)

Small Caesar salad

1 cup skim milk

Snack #1

2 reduced-fat cheese sticks with 4 whole grain crackers

Snack #2

1 ounce pistachios

Day 13

Dinner

Taco Salad (page 204)

1 cup skim milk

Snack #1

Trail Mix:
2 tablespoons dried fruit,
1 ounce peanuts or your favorite nut, and ¼ cup unsweetened cereal (like Crispix)

Snack #2

½ cup Slow Churned ice cream topped with 1 tablespoon chocolate syrup and ¼ cup sliced strawberries

Day 14

Menu Modifications

These two weeks of menus are great for everyone whose day follows a traditional pattern of waking up, sitting down, eating three meals and some snacks over the course of the day, and then going to bed. But many of us have schedules or lifestyles that don't quite fit that pattern. If that sounds familiar, then the following section is for you. Whether you work nights, work out at usual meal times, are a vegetarian, or need more or fewer calories, you'll find adjustments that you can make to the menus to fit them into your day-to-day routine.

Are You on the Road All Day?

If you're in your car all day, whether it's for work or errands, you have some different nutritional needs when trying to lose weight. Step one is to always eat a satisfying breakfast. One of the worse things you can do when you're trying to lose weight is to head out the door on an empty stomach. Probably the only thing that is worse is doing so when you'll be out driving around, with a variety of bakeries, fast-food drive-throughs, and convenience stores calling to that empty, growling belly. Selections from any of the breakfast menus here would make a good, filling start to your day.

Step two is to invest in a good-quality, lunch-sized or slightly bigger cooler, several reusable containers, and a few small icepacks. Most of the lunches and snacks in these menus are very portable; they can be packed up and brought with you on the road. This will help you eat nutritiously and not skip meals. Carrying your own meals and snacks also keeps you from the mercy of whatever restaurants or stores you happen to be near as your hunger develops.

Often, eating on the road brings with it time constraints. There is no lunch hour. If the time you have to eat is limited, you may find it easier to divide your lunch into two or more mini meals. Instead of having a meal and two snacks, you can have four or more healthy, filling snacks.

Do You Work Out in the Morning?

You've just woken up and need to get some food in your body before you exercise. Otherwise, you'll never make it past your first set of curls or your first half mile on the treadmill. However, a big breakfast may put a damper on those crunches and wind up giving you cramps on the stair machine. The solution is to have two small breakfasts: one before you hit the gym and one after. Ideally, the pre-exercise meal should be the starchy carb and fruit part, and the postexercise meal should be the protein part. For example, have some toast and fruit before and eggs after. Breakfast meals aren't always broken down quite so easily, though.

If you prefer something higher in carbs, like oatmeal, eat half before you exercise and save the rest for after, along with an extra piece of fruit for additional carbs and fluid.

If you are planning on lower-carb items, such as yogurt and fruit, make yourself some toast and have it with a glass of juice before your workout. Then enjoy the yogurt and fruit afterward. Those simple alterations to breakfast should have you exercising to the best of your ability and getting a nutritious breakfast all at the same time.

Do You Work Out During Your Lunch Hour?

Assuming you've started the day with a wholesome breakfast, your stomach isn't completely empty, but it's pretty close to it. Your best strategy is to make sure you have one of your daily snacks about an hour or so before you plan on exercising. Also, choose the one that contains that highest amount of carbohydrates. A snack based on a grain, such as bread, a bagel, popcorn, or crackers, or some yogurt with fruit would be ideal.

If you're an early riser and it's long past snack time, trying taking the fruit part of your lunch and munching on it an hour before you work out. Either of these plans will give your body some fuel to get through your workout. Then, go ahead and have your lunch (or finish your lunch) after you are done exercising.

Do You Work the Night Shift?

Working while everyone else is asleep is a unique lifestyle to get used to. A 24-hour day in your life probably looks a little bit like this: You wake up around 4:00 or 5:00 in the afternoon, get ready for work, have a meal, and head out. You're at work for eight to twelve hours, come home, maybe eat, and then head to bed. Pretty much the exact opposite of most people. But, an eating pattern to fit into that schedule isn't really too crazy and may end up being better for you than the way the rest of us eat.

Have your dinner meal at dinnertime before you go to work in the evening. This is great if you have a family. There's no need to alter any of the menu plan's dinners; all of them will work fine in this situation. When you get home from work, that's when it's time for breakfast—6:00, 7:00, 8:00 in the morning. Again, this is great if you have a family who are just starting their day. Any of the breakfasts in the menu plan will fit into an eating plan like this. So breakfast at breakfast time, dinner at dinnertime. Easy, right? Lunch is pretty easy as well. Just pack up lunch like someone who works days, and have it during your middle-of-the-night lunch break. Most of the lunches in the menu are fairly portable. Really, I think the hardest part is where to put the snacks, and a lot of that depends on how long you work. If you have a twelve-hour shift, it's probably best to bring both of your snacks to work and have one midway between arriving and lunch and the second midway between lunch and leaving. If, on the other hand, you work an eight-hour shift, you might be better off having your first snack just before you leave for work, assuming you had dinner at dinnertime, and then your second snack a couple of hours before the end of your shift.

Night shifts are notorious for having lots of junk food available. But by bringing your own food and timing your meals and snacks accordingly, you can do your job and still lose the weight you want to.

Do You Need More Calories?

Needing more calories may sound counterintuitive if you're trying to lose weight. But we all come in different sizes, and therefore we have different calorie needs, even if we're trying to lose weight. A person who is five-foot-eleven barefoot will need a lot more calories than someone who tops out at just five feet. And while you may think eating less calories just means the taller person will lose weight faster, that's not quite true. I've mentioned it earlier but it bears repeating: Cutting calories too drastically usually results in two things, and neither of them is conducive to losing weight healthfully and keeping it off. First, without enough calories and energy to survive, your body begins breaking down tissue for energy. That's actually the goal of weight loss, and as long as it is done at the right pace, fat is burned and all is well. But when you eat too little, especially in the way of carbs, your body begins burning muscle mass for energy, which is not good. In addition, not eating enough can actually slow your metabolism down, meaning you teach your body to survive on insufficient calories, which makes losing weight that much more difficult. This happens because your muscles are the parts of your body that actually do the calorie burning. If you put your body in a situation where it needs to use its own muscle, because you're not feeding it enough, you are destroying or getting rid of the part of you that actually burns calories. You're basically lowering the calorie-burning ability of your body. Bad for weight loss.

So, now that you know how important it is to eat enough, even when trying to lose weight, here are a couple of suggestions on ways you can modify the menus to help them work better for you.

- **Add an additional snack.** Look at the snacks included in the menu as well as others scattered throughout the book. These will give you ideas for what to add to a day to bump your calories up a bit.
- **Slightly increase the size of your meals.** Add some more fruit or vegetables, or try adding 50 percent more of the grain at a meal. If you're having 1 cup of spaghetti, try 1½ cups. Instead of ½ cup of rice, increase it to ¾ cup.

How do you know if you should be eating more calories? Go back to the beginning of the book and follow the steps to figure out what you need. Know that each day of the menu is right around 1,600 to 1,700 calories. If you calculate your need as greater than that, additional calories may be beneficial. Also, if you're following the menus as they're written and find yourself constantly hungry, you may need more food. Note that I'm talking about real hunger, not boredom or stress, but real stomach-growling hunger. If that's the case, try adding a bit more calories and see how you feel.

Do You Need Fewer Calories?

Before you start cutting out food willy-nilly, figure out a rough idea of how many calories you should be eating to lose weight. Go to Part 1 in the front of the book and find the section on determining your calorie needs. Follow the steps to figure out what you need, keeping in mind you shouldn't be eating fewer than 1,300 or so calories a day to stay healthy. If your calculations result in fewer than 1,300 calories to promote weight loss, your safest, healthiest bet is to increase your exercise to make up for the additional calories. For example, if you determine that losing weight requires you to eat 1,100 calories a day, you should eat 1,300 but exercise more to burn off the extra 200 calories each day. Make sense?

But if you do need to eat fewer calories, one simple step is to cut out one snack. Depending on the snack, that will decrease your intake by anywhere from about 150 to 200 calories a day. Find you really like both of those snacks? No problem. Cut each in half. They'll still give you a little between-meal nibble, but overall you'll be taking in fewer calories. Another way to go about it is to decrease your meal size by just a little. Usually the grain group is the group with which you have the most wiggle room. So instead of a whole English muffin, try half. Instead of 1 cup of pasta, try ¾ cup. You could apply the same to starchy veggies. Instead of a medium potato, have a small one.

One by one they may seem like small changes, which will make them easier to keep up with, but they can really add up over the course of a week or a month. Just 300 fewer calories a day equals a pound lost in about a week and a half. Again, that may not seem like much, but that's about thirty-five pounds a year. Then add on to that the calories cut or burned and pounds lost from exercising and other changes, such as cutting out sugary drinks and so forth. You can see how easily small, simple changes can really make a difference.

Are You a Vegetarian?

If you're following a vegetarian diet, these menus should be fairly easy to convert. For breakfast, if you're a lacto-ovo vegetarian, you don't need to make any changes. None of the breakfasts include meat of any kind. If you do not eat dairy products, you can easily swap the milk, yogurt, and cheese found in the breakfast recipes with soy milk, yogurt, and cheese. If you eat dairy but not eggs, there are only two breakfasts containing eggs in the two weeks of menus. Feel free to replace them with other, more appealing breakfasts from the two-week period.

There are six lunches on the menu that already do not include meat. If you eat seafood, you can add three more lunches to the list of ones you needn't change. As for the remaining five meals, several would be equally nutritious, calorie conscious, and delicious if you were to replace the meat with soy crumbles, soy dogs, soy burgers, or even tofu. Also, if you especially enjoy one or two of the recommended lunches, you can double up on them to replace other meat-containing meals.

With regards to dinner, four are already meatless. The Thai Noodles would be equally delicious without the shrimp, and there is one other salmon dinner if you still eat seafood. The meatloaf, tacos, and taco salad are all ideal recipes in which to use soy crumbles or one of the various meatless ground beef alternatives by companies such as Morningstar Farms. Soy chicken strips can be heated and sauced or seasoned similarly to the chicken breast in the appropriate recipes. And, if you find that there are still meals that don't appeal to you, go ahead and replace them with duplicates or even leftovers from meals you did like.

When it comes to snacks, many are fine as is, but you could add soy nuts to your list of possible snacks as a crunchy way to boost your protein intake. And of course if you don't consume dairy foods, the milk, ice cream, cheeses, and yogurts can all be replaced easily with soy alternatives with no negative impact on your calorie intake or weight.

when to
eat what
recipes

All of these recipes can be doubled or halved easily.

Each recipe includes nutrition information.

Southwest Scramble

INGREDIENTS | Serves 1

2 large eggs

1 tablespoon reduced-fat shredded Mexican blend or Cheddar cheese

1 diced jalapeño pepper

2 tablespoons diced or grated onion

Heat a small nonstick skillet over medium-low heat. In small bowl, whisk eggs until well blended. Pour into heated skillet and cook, stirring often, until eggs are almost set. Sprinkle on remaining ingredients and stir until well combined and heated through. Serve.

Calories: 181 | Protein: 15 grams | Carbohydrates: 4 grams | Fiber: <1 gram | Total Fat: 12 grams | Saturated Fat: 4 grams | Sodium: 281 milligrams

Ham Roll Up

INGREDIENTS | Serves 1

1 whole wheat tortilla (1.5 ounce)

1 teaspoon honey mustard

2 ounces thinly sliced, reduced-sodium deli ham

½ cup shredded or chopped romaine lettuce

Spread tortilla with honey mustard. Top with ham and lettuce. Roll up and enjoy.

Calories: 238 | Protein: 17 grams | Carbohydrates: 22 grams | Fiber: 2 grams | Total Fat: 7 grams | Saturated Fat: 2 grams | Sodium: 725 milligrams

when to eat what

Italian Meatloaf

INGREDIENTS | Serves 5

1 pound lean ground beef (93% lean)

¾ cup oats

1 teaspoon dried oregano

1 teaspoon dried basil

1 teaspoon onion powder

1 egg

1 cup reduced-sodium marinara/
spaghetti sauce, divided in half

¼ cup reduced-fat shredded
mozzarella cheese

Dash of salt

Dash of pepper

Preheat oven to 350°F. In medium bowl, combine all ingredients except ½ cup marinara sauce, and mix well. Place in a nonstick loaf pan. Bake for 1 hour, until done. While baking, brush with remaining marinara sauce every 15 minutes, until it reaches an internal temperature of 165°F.

Calories: 233 | Protein: 23 grams | Carbohydrates: 16 grams | Fiber: 3 grams | Total Fat: 8 grams | Saturated Fat: 3 grams | Sodium: 136 milligrams

Blueberry Cobbler Oatmeal

INGREDIENTS | Serves 1

1 packet plain instant oatmeal

1 cup skim milk, divided into ⅔ and ⅓

3 tablespoons frozen blueberries

¼ teaspoon vanilla

Dash cinnamon

Combine oatmeal, ⅔ cup milk, blueberries, vanilla, and cinnamon in a microwave-safe bowl. Heat, uncovered, on HIGH for 1 minute. Stir, heat 1 minute more. Stir again and continue heating in 30-second increments until it reaches the desired consistency. Serve with remaining ⅓ cup milk.

Calories: 200 | Protein: 12 grams | Carbohydrates: 35 grams | Fiber: 4 grams | Total Fat: 2 grams | Saturated Fat: 0 grams | Sodium: 183 milligrams

Crunchy Tuna Salad

INGREDIENTS | Serves 2

6-ounce can water-packed tuna, drained

3 teaspoons reduced-fat mayonnaise

2 tablespoons grated, shredded, or finely chopped carrot

2 tablespoons slivered almonds

Combine all ingredients in a bowl and mix well. Eat immediately or chill for up to 24 hours until ready to serve.

Calories: 157 | Protein: 21 grams | Carbohydrates: 3 grams | Fiber: 1 gram | Total Fat: 7 grams | Saturated Fat: 1 gram | Sodium: 440 milligrams

Quick Mexican Pizza

INGREDIENTS | Serves 1

⅓ cup fat-free refried beans

1 whole wheat tortilla (1.5 ounce)

2 tablespoons reduced-fat shredded Mexican blend or Cheddar cheese

2 tablespoons shredded lettuce

2 tablespoons diced tomato

2 teaspoons reduced-fat sour cream

This can be eaten warm or cold.

For warm, preheat oven to 350°F. Spread beans evenly over tortilla. Top with cheese, lettuce, and tomato. Place on baking sheet in preheated oven and bake just until it is heated through and cheese melts, about 10 minutes. Top with sour cream and cut into wedges.

To eat cold, top with sour cream and cut into wedges or roll up. There is no need to bake it first.

Calories: 251 | Protein: 12 grams | Carbohydrates: 34 grams | Fiber: 6 grams | Total Fat: 7 grams | Saturated Fat: 3 grams | Sodium: 639 milligrams

Really Big Salad

INGREDIENTS | Serves 1

1½ cups baby spinach

1½ cups romaine lettuce, chopped

½ medium cucumber, sliced

1 medium tomato, diced

¼ cup shredded carrots

2 thin slices red onion

1 hardboiled egg, chopped

2 tablespoons reduced-fat shredded Cheddar cheese

1 tablespoon shelled sunflower seeds

2 tablespoons reduced-fat French dressing

Combine first six ingredients. Top with egg, cheese, and seeds. Serve with dressing on the side.

Calories: 361 | Protein: 17 grams | Carbohydrates: 34 grams | Fiber: 8 grams | Total Fat: 19 grams | Saturated Fat: 4 grams | Sodium: 578 milligrams

Breakfast Banana Split

INGREDIENTS | Serves 1

1 medium banana, sliced lengthwise

⅓ cup nonfat strawberry yogurt

⅓ cup nonfat vanilla yogurt

2 tablespoons chopped walnuts

Place 1 medium banana, sliced lengthwise in a bowl. Top with ⅓ cup nonfat strawberry yogurt and ⅓ cup nonfat vanilla yogurt. Sprinkle with 2 tablespoons chopped walnuts.

Calories: 332 | Protein: 10 grams | Carbohydrates: 55 grams | Fiber: 4 grams | Total Fat: 11 grams | Saturated Fat: 1 gram | Sodium: 99 milligrams

when to eat *what*

Grilled Salmon

INGREDIENTS | Serves 2

½ cup light teriyaki sauce

½ cup water

½ pound boneless salmon fillets

1 tablespoon canola oil

Mix teriyaki sauce and water in a medium bowl. Place fish in bowl and marinate for 10 minutes.

Heat oil in a grill pan over medium heat or brush grill rack with oil. Grill 4 to 5 minutes on each side until fish flakes easily with a fork.

Calories: 313 | Protein: 24 grams | Carbohydrates: 3 grams | Fiber: 0 grams | Total Fat: 22 grams | Saturated Fat: 4 grams | Sodium: 387 milligrams

Lemon-Infused Couscous

INGREDIENTS | Serves 1

¼ cup plain couscous

¼ cup chicken stock

½ teaspoon olive oil

Zest of half a lemon

Following package directions, prepare coucous using stock, oil, and lemon zest in place of ingredients listed on package.

Calories: 122 | Protein: 5 grams | Carbohydrates: 22 grams | Fiber: 1 gram | Total Fat: 3 grams | Saturated Fat: < 1 gram | Sodium: 108 milligrams

Pan-Fried Italian Chicken

INGREDIENTS | Serves 2

1½ tablespoons olive oil

2 (4-ounce) chicken breasts

1½ teaspoons salt-free
Italian seasoning

Heat oil in nonstick skillet over medium heat.

While oil heats, pound chicken breasts to an even thickness, about ½". Rub seasoning on both sides of chicken.

Place chicken in heated skillet. Cook about 5 to 6 minutes on first side. Turn and cook an additional 4 to 5 minutes, or until chicken has reached an internal temperature of 165°F.

Calories: 215 | Protein: 25 grams | Carbohydrates: 0 grams | Fiber: 0 grams | Total Fat: 12 grams | Saturated Fat: 2 grams | Sodium: 56 milligrams

when to eat *what*

Roasted Red Potatoes and Broccoli

INGREDIENTS | Serves 2

½ pound small red potatoes

¼ pound broccoli florets

1 tablespoon olive oil

¼ teaspoon kosher salt

Dash of black pepper

1 clove garlic, minced or grated

Heat oven to 400°F.

Cut the potatoes in halves or quarters. Cut broccoli in bite-sized pieces. Place potatoes and broccoli in bowl with olive oil, salt, pepper, and garlic. Mix until well coated.

Spread potatoes in a single layer on a large, rimmed, baking sheet. Roast in preheated oven for 35 minutes.

Remove from oven and flip potatoes. Add broccoli and return to oven to continue roasting for about 20 to 25 more minutes, until potatoes are browned and crisp and broccoli is softened and lightly browned. Stir once or twice during final roasting.

Calories: 186 | Protein: 4 grams | Carbohydrates: 27 grams | Fiber: 4 grams | Total Fat: 7 grams | Saturated Fat: 1 gram | Sodium: 277 milligrams

Cinnamon Popcorn

INGREDIENTS | Serves 1

3 cups freshly popped plain air-popped or light microwave popcorn

2 teaspoons tub/spreadable margarine

1 teaspoon sugar

¼ teaspoon cinnamon

While popcorn is still hot, immediately stir in margarine, sugar, and cinnamon. Shake well to combine.

Calories: 77 | Protein: 3 grams | Carbohydrates: 23 grams | Fiber: 4 grams | Total Fat: 9 grams | Saturated Fat: 1 gram | Sodium: 64 milligrams

Salmon-Topped Salad

INGREDIENTS | Serves 1

1½ cups chopped romaine lettuce

½ medium tomato, chopped

¼ medium cucumber, sliced

2 tablespoons shredded carrots

3 ounces canned salmon

2 tablespoons reduced-fat balsamic vinaigrette

Combine first four ingredients. Top with salmon. Drizzle with vinaigrette.

Calories: 213 | Protein: 18 grams | Carbohydrates: 12 grams | Fiber: 3 grams | Total Fat: 11 grams | Saturated Fat: 1 gram | Sodium: 702 milligrams

when to eat what

Apple Burrito

INGREDIENTS | Serves 1

1 whole wheat tortilla (1.5 ounce)

1 tablespoon crunchy peanut butter

1 small apple, chopped

1 teaspoon honey

Spread tortilla with peanut butter. Sprinkle apples on top. Drizzle with honey. Roll up. Slice in half if desired.

Calories: 320 | Protein: 8 grams | Carbohydrates: 50 grams | Fiber: 6 grams | Total Fat: 11 grams | Saturated Fat: 2 grams | Sodium: 221 milligrams

Turkey Pita

INGREDIENTS | Serves 1

One 6½" whole wheat pita

2 teaspoons mustard

2 ounces thinly sliced low-sodium, deli-style turkey

2 tomato slices

Spread pita with mustard. Fill pita with turkey and tomato slices.

Calories: 234 | Protein: 20 grams | Carbohydrates: 39 grams | Fiber: 6 grams | Total Fat: 2 grams | Saturated Fat: < 1 gram | Sodium: 880 milligrams

Soft Turkey Tacos

INGREDIENTS | Serves 4

1 pound 99% fat-free ground turkey

2 teaspoons cumin

2 tablespoons chili powder

1 teaspoon garlic powder

½ teaspoon onion powder

½ cup water

8 tablespoons reduced-fat, shredded Cheddar cheese

8 (1½-ounce) whole wheat flour tortillas

Optional toppings: shredded lettuce, chopped tomato, salsa

Brown turkey in nonstick skillet, breaking up chunks with spoon as it cooks. Drain fat, if any. Add spices and water. Cover and simmer 5 to 10 minutes.

To serve, divide meat and cheese evenly between tortillas. Top with desired toppings.

Calories: 426 | Protein: 39 grams | Carbohydrates: 41 grams | Fiber: 4 grams | Total Fat: 11 grams | Saturated Fat: 2 grams | Sodium: 466 milligrams

when to eat *what*

Sunshine Smoothie

INGREDIENTS | Serves 1

½ cup nonfat plain yogurt

½ cup 100% orange juice

1 small sliced frozen banana

Combine all in a blender and blend until well combined and little to no chunks remain.

Calories: 196 | Protein: 7 grams | Carbohydrates: 46 grams | Fiber: 3 grams | Total Fat: 1 gram | Saturated Fat: 0 grams | Sodium: 70 milligrams

Nut-n-Honey Sandwich

INGREDIENTS | Serves 1

1½ tablespoons peanut butter

2 slices cinnamon bread

2 teaspoons honey

Spread peanut butter evenly on each slice of bread. Drizzle honey on top of peanut butter and spread. Top one slice of bread with other, peanut butter sides together.

Calories: 345 | Protein: 12 grams | Carbohydrates: 45 grams | Fiber: 4 grams | Total Fat: 15 grams | Saturated Fat: 2 grams | Sodium: 323 milligrams

Ham and Sweet Potato Skillet

INGREDIENTS | Serves 2

2 medium sweet potatoes

1½ teaspoons butter

¼ cup 100% orange juice

2 tablespoons packed light brown sugar

6 ounces low-sodium ham steak or leftover ham

Bake potatoes in oven or microwave until tender. Let cool slightly then peel and cut into bite-sized chunks. In a large skillet, heat butter just until melted. Add orange juice and brown sugar and stir to dissolve sugar. Heat to a simmer. Add ham and sweet potatoes just to heat through.

Calories: 347 | Protein: 21 grams | Carbohydrates: 44 grams | Fiber: 4 grams | Total Fat: 10 grams | Saturated Fat: 4 grams | Sodium: 896 milligrams

California Egg Salad Sandwich

INGREDIENTS | Serves 1

1 large egg

2 slices whole grain bread

½ teaspoon reduced-fat mayonnaise

1 tablespoon mashed, ripe avocado

Hard boil egg. Let cool slightly, then peel. While egg cooks, toast bread. Once egg is peeled, place it in a small bowl along with mayonnaise and avocado. Using a fork, mash until well combined and only a few small chunks remain. Spread egg mixture on one piece of toast. Top with remaining toast.

Calories: 289 | Protein: 15 grams | Carbohydrates: 32 grams | Fiber: 7 grams | Total Fat: 12 grams | Saturated Fat: 2 grams | Sodium: 383 milligrams

when to eat what

Chicken Scampi

INGREDIENTS | Serves 2

1 tablespoon olive oil

1 tablespoon butter

2 cups sliced red pepper (about 2 medium peppers)

6-ounce boneless, skinless chicken breast, cut into bite-sized pieces

¼ cup white wine

¼ cup chicken stock

2 tablespoons lemon juice

Heat olive oil and butter in a large skillet over medium heat. Add peppers and sauté until tender-crisp. Add chicken pieces and continue cooking about 8 minutes, until chicken is cooked through. Add wine, stock, and lemon juice and simmer 3 to 4 minutes.

Calories: 272 | Protein: 19 grams | Carbohydrates: 10 grams | Fiber: 2 grams | Total Fat: 15 grams | Saturated Fat: 5 grams | Sodium: 147 milligrams

Breakfast Sandwich

INGREDIENTS | Serves 1

1 whole grain English muffin

1 egg

1 tablespoon reduced-fat, shredded Cheddar cheese

1 slice tomato

Toast English muffin. While muffin toasts, scramble egg in a small, nonstick skillet. Stir in cheese just until it melts. Remove from heat. Layer egg and tomato slice between 'muffin halves.

Calories: 196 | Protein: 13 grams | Carbohydrates: 27 grams | Fiber: 9 grams | Total Fat: 8 grams | Saturated Fat: 3 grams | Sodium: 276 milligrams

Crab Melt

INGREDIENTS | Serves 1

3 ounces canned crab

1½ teaspoons reduced-fat mayonnaise

1 whole wheat English muffin, toasted

2 slices tomato

1½ tablespoons reduced-fat, shredded Cheddar cheese

Preheat oven or toaster oven to broil. Combine crab and mayo. Spread evenly on muffin halves. Place a tomato slice on each muffin. Sprinkle cheese evenly over tomatoes. Place under broiler until cheese melts.

Calories: 268 | Protein: 23 grams | Carbohydrates: 29 grams | Fiber: 9 grams | Total Fat: 11 grams | Saturated Fat: 2 grams | Sodium: 698 grams

Rice and Beans

INGREDIENTS | Serves 2

1½ tablespoons olive oil

2 tablespoons chopped onion

1 clove garlic, minced or grated

½ medium red or green pepper, chopped

1 tablespoon tomato paste

Dash of cayenne pepper

1 cup canned small red beans, drained and rinsed

½ cup uncooked white rice

1¼ cups water

Heat oil in a large skillet over medium heat. Add onion, garlic, pepper, paste, and cayenne. Sauté until onion and pepper are tender. Add beans, rice, and water. Heat to boil, and then simmer, covered, until water is absorbed and rice is cooked, about 20 minutes.

Calories: 463 | Protein: 12 grams | Carbohydrates: 76 grams | Fiber: 9 grams | Total Fat: 12 grams | Saturated Fat: 2 grams | Sodium: 39 milligrams

when to eat what

Rum Raisin Oatmeal

INGREDIENTS | Serves 1

1 packet plain instant oatmeal

1 cup skim milk, divided into ⅔ and ⅓

2 tablespoons raisins

¼ teaspoon rum extract

Dash cinnamon

Combine oatmeal, ⅔ cup milk, raisins, rum extract, and cinnamon in a microwave-safe bowl. Heat, uncovered, on HIGH for 1 minute. Stir, heat 1 minute more. Stir again and continue heating in 30-second increments until it reaches the desired consistency. Serve with remaining ⅓ cup milk.

Calories: 248 | Protein: 13 grams | Carbohydrates: 47 grams | Fiber: 4 grams | Total Fat: 2 grams | Saturated Fat: 0 grams | Sodium: 188 milligrams

English Muffin Pizza

INGREDIENTS | Serves 1

2 tablespoons pizza or spaghetti sauce

1 whole grain English muffin, split

3 tablespoons reduced-fat, shredded mozzarella cheese

Preheat oven or toaster oven to 375°F. Spread sauce evenly on muffin halves; top with cheese. Bake for about 10 minutes, until cheese is melted.

Calories: 180 | Protein: 12 grams | Carbohydrates: 31 grams | Fiber: 10 grams | Total Fat: 5 grams | Saturated Fat: 2 grams | Sodium: 320 milligrams

Thai Shrimp Noodles

INGREDIENTS | Serves 2

4 ounces whole wheat spaghetti

2 teaspoons canola oil

1 medium red pepper cut into short, thick strips

2 tablespoons water

2 tablespoons peanut butter

1 tablespoon reduced-sodium soy sauce

½ tablespoon cider vinegar

Dash of cayenne pepper

1 teaspoon honey

½ pound peeled, cooked shrimp

Cook pasta according to package directions. In small skillet, heat oil over medium heat and sauté red peppers until tender. In small saucepot, combine next 6 ingredients and heat, stirring occasionally, until smooth. Combine cooked and drained pasta, peppers, sauce, and shrimp. Mix well. Serve.

Calories: 455 | Protein: 32 grams | Carbohydrates: 54 grams | Fiber: 9 grams | Total Fat: 15 grams | Saturated Fat: 2 grams | Sodium: 528 milligrams

Grilled Chicken

INGREDIENTS | Serves 1

1 5-oz boneless, skinless chicken breast

½ tsp olive oil

Salt-free seasoning

Brush chicken breast with olive oil and sprinkle with your favorite salt-free seasoning.

Grill or broil until cooked through and chicken has reached an internal temperature of 165°F.

Calories: 173 | Protein: 29 grams | Carbohydrates: 0 grams | Fiber: 0 grams | Total Fat: 6 grams | Saturated Fat: 1 grams | Sodium: 68 milligrams

when to eat what

Spicy Popcorn

INGREDIENTS | Serves 1

3 cups freshly popped plain air-popped or light microwave popcorn

2 teaspoons tub/spreadable margarine

1 teaspoon chili powder

While popcorn is still hot, immediately stir in margarine and chili powder. Shake well to combine.

Calories: 169 | Protein: 3 grams | Carbohydrates: 20 grams | Fiber: 4 grams | Total Fat: 9 grams | Saturated Fat: 2 grams | Sodium: 90 milligrams

Roast Beef Sandwich

INGREDIENTS | Serves 1

2 teaspoons reduced-fat mayonnaise

2 slices whole grain bread

2 ounces thinly sliced, low-sodium, deli-style roast beef

1-ounce slice Cheddar cheese

Spread mayonnaise on each slice of bread. Top one slice, mayonnaise side, with roast beef and cheese. Place remaining slice of bread on top of cheese, mayonnaise-side down.

Calories: 355 | Protein: 28 grams | Carbohydrates: 29 grams | Fiber: 8 grams | Total Fat: 14 grams | Saturated Fat: 6 grams | Sodium: 492 milligrams

Taco Salad

INGREDIENTS | Serves 6

1 pound 93% lean ground beef, cooked and drained

3 medium tomatoes, chopped

½ head iceberg lettuce, chopped or shredded

1 cup (4 ounces) reduced-fat, shredded Cheddar cheese

6-ounce bag baked tortilla chips, crushed

½ cup reduced-fat Italian dressing

½ cup reduced-fat Ranch dressing

Combine first five ingredients in a large bowl. Mix dressings and stir into salad.

Calories: 397 | Protein: 30 grams | Carbohydrates: 34 grams | Fiber: 3 grams | Total Fat: 17 grams | Saturated Fat: 5 grams | Sodium: 789 milligrams

when to eat what

appendix a

resource list

websites

American Dietetic Association
www.eatright.org

> Tips about healthy eating, food and nutrition information, how to find a registered dietitian in your area, and more.

My Pyramid (United States Department of Agriculture)
www.MyPyramid.gov

> Log on to get more information about MyPyramid and to personalize it for you and your family.

National Dairy Council
www.nationaldairycouncil.org

> Nutrition information, recipes, and more about a variety of dairy foods.

Nutrition.gov
www.nutrition.gov

> Information on nutrition, healthy eating, food safety, and more.

Produce for Better Health Foundation
www.fruitsandveggiesmorematters.org

> Nutrition information, tips, recipes, and more about fruits and vegetables.

Supermarket Savvy
www.supermarketsavvy.com

> Information on healthier grocery shopping.

when to eat what

U.S. Department of Health & Human Services

www.healthierus.gov/dietaryguidelines

The most current Dietary Guidelines for Americans, and related articles.

101 Foods That Could Save Your Life

www.101foodsthatcouldsaveyourlife.com

Video library of 101 healthy foods.

newsletters

Environmental Nutrition

www.environmentalnutrition.com

Each issue provides, among other things, updates on current nutrition research, cutting-edge reports on a variety of nutrition topics, and a nutrition comparison helping you make the best food choices in the supermarket and restaurants to benefit your health.

Nutrition Action Health Letter

www.cspinet.org/nah/index.htm

The popular newsletter from The Center for Science in the Public Interest (CSPI) provides consumers with current and useful information about their health and well-being by educating them on the foods and drinks available to them on a regular basis.

Tufts University Health and Nutrition Letter

www.healthletter.tufts.edu

Reliable, trusted, and scientifically accurate health and nutrition advice based largely on the research and expertise of the Tufts University Gerald J. and Dorothy R. Friedman School of Nutrition Science and Policy.

appendix b

pantry items

For quick, easy, and healthy eating, you need to start with an arsenal of nutritious ingredients. This section lists some foods and ingredients that you should keep on hand so you're never at a loss for a healthy meal.

Grains

- Whole grain or 100% whole wheat bread
- Whole grain pitas
- Whole grain tortillas
- Whole grain English muffins
- Regular and whole wheat pasta—different shapes and sizes
- Oats
- Plain instant oatmeal packets
- Whole grain cereals such as Total, Life, Fiber One, or Cheerios

Dairy

- Skim or 1% low-fat milk
- Reduced-fat sour cream
- Reduced-fat shredded cheese
- Plain and/or vanilla low-fat, or nonfat Greek yogurt

Protein

- Canned beans (low-sodium if possible)
- Peanut butter
- Nuts (a variety, such as peanuts, almonds, walnuts, cashews, pistachios)
- Boneless, skinless chicken breasts
- Water-packed tuna
- Canned salmon
- Eggs

Produce

- Fresh fruits and vegetables (buy a small amount each week to prevent spoilage and waste)
- Frozen fruit (without added sauces or syrups)
- Frozen vegetables (without added sauces or seasonings)
- Salsa
- Low-sodium tomato sauce
- Low-sodium pasta sauce
- Canned fruits (canned in juice, not syrup)
- Dried fruits (a variety, such as raisins, blueberries, cranberries, cherries, apricots)

Other Staples

- Olive oil
- Canola oil
- Nonstick cooking spray
- Chicken stock
- Beef stock
- Vegetable stock
- Low-sodium soups
- Reduced-fat salad dressings

index

Note: Page numbers in **bold** indicate recipes.

Afternoon. *See* Night/late afternoon scenarios; Noon/afternoon scenarios
Alcohol
    affecting calorie consumption, 48, 68–69
    beer, 96
    benefits of, 18, 96
    calories by type of drink, 96–97
    designated driver and, 119
    drinks to keep weight in check and to avoid, 96–97
    eating before having, 128
    happy hour considerations, 118–19
    keeping you awake, 40
    late dinner and, 55
    liquor, 97
    before vs. during meals, 48, 68–69
    reducing effects of, 68–69
    sobering up after, 128
    stimulating appetite, 48
    wine, 96–97
Antioxidants
    in fruit, 63, 66
    minimizing environmental damage, 62
    in salad greens, 114, 157–58
    supplements, 92
Apple Burrito, **195**

Baby weight, losing, 125–29
Bananas
    about: potassium from, 4, 18, 143; with yogurt for breakfast, 18
    Breakfast Banana Split, **190**
Barbecues, food options, 53–54
Barbell icon. *See* Working-out scenarios

Beans and legumes
    about: as protein source, 87–88
    Quick Mexican Pizza, **189**
    Rice and Beans, **200**
Beef. *See* Meat; Meat recipes
Beer, 96
Beverages. *See also* Alcohol
    afternoon coffee drinks, 16–17
    brown-bag options, 161
    coffee before workouts, 36
    for hiking, 19
    sleep problems and, 39
    staying hydrated, 19
    Sunshine Smoothie, **197**
Blood sugar. *See also* Diabetes
    fruits and, 32–33
    headaches, hypoglycemia and, 154–55
Blueberry Cobbler Oatmeal, **188**
Body mass index (BMI), 7, 94
Breads. *See also* Pizza
    about: English muffin for breakfast, 18; enjoying and controlling portions, 137–38; toast for breakfast, 90
    Pumpkin Pancakes, **110**
Breakfast
    after overeating last night, 104
    balanced, easy-to-go options, 18
    benefits of, 18, 85, 148
    best ways to prepare eggs, 74–75
    brunch and, 77, 135
    calories per meal, 77
    cereal contents and portion sizes, 85
    decent-sized, 77
    for delicate stomachs, 99
    fiber and protein for, 62, 148
    forgetting to eat, 90
    fruits and, 41, 62
    healthy frozen dishes, 52

when to eat *what*

when to eat *what*

when to eat *what*

when to eat *what*

about the author

Heidi Reichenberger McIndoo, MS, RD, LDN, is a nutrition consultant, spokesperson, and author who has been a registered dietitian for eighteen years and worked for more than twelve years as an outpatient dietitian at a small hospital and a community health center. She has contributed to numerous health-related books and magazines, including *Prevention, Eating Light, Family Circle, Shape,* and more, and has been the national spokesperson for companies such as VitaminWater. She lives in Boston, Massachusetts.